SICKNESS: ITS TRIALS AND BLESSINGS

By Priscilla Maurice

The Christian Classic on Chronic Illness in Modern English

Edited and updated by
Alison Bailey Castellina

Tempo di Riforma
Publications
2009

Sickness: its Trials and Blessings

> There are varieties of gifts, but the same Spirit.
>
> For the body does not consist of one member but of many.
>
> But as it is, God arranged the members in the body, each one of them, as he chose.
>
> If one member suffers, all suffer together; if one member is honoured, all rejoice together.
>
> (1 Corinthians 12:4,24,26)

This volume is affectionately dedicated to all who are called by sickness to walk in the blessed steps of His most holy life, who Himself bore our sickness.

Priscilla Maurice, 1850.

ISBN: 9781409279327

The text used for this modernised edition is the 5th edition by Rivingtons, Waterloo Place, London which was published in 1855.

"Unless otherwise indicated, all Scripture quotations are from The Holy Bible, English Standard Version, published by HarperCollinsPublishers ©2001 by Crossway Bibles, a division of Good News Publishers. Used by permission. All rights reserved."

This work is licensed under the Creative Commons Attribution-No Derivative Works 2.0 UK: England & Wales License. To view a copy of this license, visit http://creativecommons.org/licenses/by-nd/2.0/uk/ or send a letter to Creative Commons, 171 Second Street, Suite 300, San Francisco, California, 94105, USA.

The editor Alison Bailey Castellina can be contacted by email at the address **baileyannis@googlemail.com**. See also her website at http://fatigue.wikispaces.com

Sickness: its Trials and Blessings

Table of Contents

Preface..7
    BACKGROUND...7
    EDITORIAL TECHNIQUE...12
    A GIFT TO THE SICK..14
    BIOGRAPHICAL NOTE ON PRISCILLA MAURICE........................15
    PREFACE BY A MINISTER OF RELIGION (1850)............................27

Part I - New Ways of Looking at Illness.......................29
    INTRODUCTION...29
    1.1 FIRST IMPRESSIONS OF A LONG ILLNESS OR CHRONIC CONDITION..34
    1.2 ILLNESS: A HIDDEN STATE..36
    1.3 THE TWOFOLD CHARACTER OF ILLNESS...............................39
    1.4 THE SEEMING LENGTH OF AN ILLNESS................................40
    1.5 LESSONS WHICH VARIOUS ILLNESSES ARE MEANT TO TEACH........42
    1.6 SICKNESS AS A VOCATION..44
    1.7 THE PROBABILITY OF RECOVERY...48

Part II - ASPECTS OF ILLNESS..51
    2.1 PAIN...51
    2.2 WEAKNESS...54
    The Variation of Weakness in Different People..............55
    The Problem of Sensitivity to Light................................56
    The Problem of Sensitivity to External Noises.................57
    The Habits of Illness...57
    Weakness of Mind..58
    Mental and Spiritual Warfare..58

- *Resisting the Devil in Illness*...*59*
- *Evil Desires in Illness*..*60*
- *Getting confused in what you say*...............................*61*
- *The Unknown and Foreign Nature of Illness*................*61*
- 2.3 LOSS OF THE POWERS OF THE MIND..65
  - *Grief over Mental Losses in Illness*..............................*67*
  - *Loss of Memory*..*67*
  - *Inability to Talk*..*70*
- 2.4 THE NEARNESS OF LIFE..72
- 2.5 LONGINGS...73
- 2.6 CIRCUMSTANCES...77
- 2.7 WHAT EFFORT TO MAKE AND HOW TO ACHIEVE SELF CONTROL......81
- 2.8 IRRITABLE NERVES...86
- 2.9 TAKING DRUGS..90
- 2.10 LONGING FOR FOOD..92
  - *Fasting*..*94*
  - *The Blessing of Social and Communal Meals*..............*95*
  - *Eating Alone*...*95*
- 2.11 NIGHTS...96
- 2.12 DAYS..99
  - *Choice of Reading Matter*..*101*
- 2.13 DISAPPOINTMENTS AND DISCOURAGEMENTS..........................105
- 2.14 WORRIES ABOUT LACK OF MONEY IN ILLNESS.........................107
- 2.15 DIFFICULTY IN PRAYER...110
- 2.16 ABSENCE OF WORK..122
- 2.17 ANNIVERSARIES...126

2.18 FAMILY AND FRIENDS..131
2.19 LETTERS AND COMMUNICATIONS.................................139
2.20 VISITS OF THE CLERGY AND CHRISTIAN MINISTERS..............141
2.21 MEDICAL ADVICE AND MEDICAL VISITS.........................146
2.22 NURSES AND CARERS..152
2.23 BEING A BURDEN..157
2.24 THE TEMPTATION TO THINK THAT NO ONE CAN SYMPATHIZE.....159
2.25 IRRITABILITY..161
2.26 IMPATIENCE...164
2.27 CONSIDERING SYMPTOMS..165

PART III - DUTIES AND RESPONSIBILITIES OF ILLNESS 167

3.1 CONTENTMENT...167
Sin towards God *170*
Sin towards your neighbour *170*
Sin against yourself *171*
3.2 SYMPATHY..174
3.2 PATIENCE...179
3.4 SUBMISSION...185
3.5 HOPE..192
5.6 CHEERFULNESS..196
5.7 THANKSGIVING..202
3.8 TO REMEMBER THOSE IN NEED AND TO HELP OTHERS..............208

Part IV - THE BLESSINGS OF ILLNESS.......................211

Part V - MISCELLANEOUS..219

5.1 READING THE SCRIPTURES..219

5.2 Sunday, the Lord's Day..220

5.3 The Lord's Supper..228

5.4 Prayer for Healing..233

Part VI - CONVALESCENCE..237

6.1 Its pleasures and Its trials...237

6.2 Being Called Back to Life - how to Accept Life Again.....241

Part VII - DEATH..247

7.1 The fear of death - the fear of it taken away.................247

7.2 A public death-bed, and the desire to choose its circumstances 251

7.3 The Right Way of Viewing Death 253

APPENDIX 257

Suggestions to those ministering to the sick and dying...........257

THE ORDER FOR THE VISITATION OF THE SICK........263

A Prayer for a sick Child..270

A Prayer for a sick person, when there appeareth small hope of recovery. 270

A commendatory Prayer for a sick person at the point of departure..271

A Prayer for persons troubled in mind or in conscience 272

The Communion of the Sick..272

Sickness: its Trials and Blessings

Preface

Background

The author of this best-selling book, which was first published in 1850, remained unidentified to her readers. Her name never appeared on the covers of any of her books.

It has been my desire, ever since I first read this book, twenty years ago, to discover more about the author and to restore her name to its deserved place on the front cover. Our edition has embedded the full Bible texts within the body of the text and has added, for the first time, a short biography of its writer, Priscilla Maurice.

Who was Priscilla Maurice? How could someone ill handle the Bible so comprehensively? What was her purpose in writing? How did she develop her writing skills? These are some of the questions that I tried to answer.

After research, I was not surprised to find that Priscilla Maurice was the sister of leading Victorian and Cambridge don, Frederick Denison Maurice (F. D. Maurice), co-founder with Charles Kingsley, of Christian Socialism, author, editor of the forerunner of the New Statesman magazine, Anglican minister and Cambridge professor. He was hailed by the British Prime Minister, Gladstone as a 'spiritual splendour'.

Like her brother, Priscilla Maurice was gifted with skills as a writer, deep compassion and a burning desire to serve mankind. But she added to these abilities one which, I believe, is the reason why this book still is relevant today. She had a deep love for the Bible which she had read in a way that only a few scholars today could rival. It is the Bible's depth that does makes this book just a relevant now, as it was when it was first published.

Sickness: its Trials and Blessings

Learned and literary, Priscilla Maurice wrote at many levels. She could pursue a 'good work' on behalf of others, bring to light deep doctrine and also give a most fascinating insight into what Victorian life was like for an unmarried woman with well married sisters, enduring a long and misunderstood illness. One of the joys of this book is that it is a kind of time capsule, of interest to those who enjoy the flavour of the Victorian age.

I believe that for the author, the experience of having had her own faith and life stripped of what she calls its 'gloss', preserved in her, particularly, a very precious strand of holy fire, a kind of testament about the power of the Bible in the 'religious' Victorian age. She undoubtedly saw herself as one of those who in health and sickness wanted "to work for the lasting good of the Church, as well as for this sick member[1]". Yet even she might be surprised that people are still finding her book relevant, over 150 years after it was published.

On another level, Priscilla Maurice felt called to write with powerful eloquence on behalf of the sick, to describe and to reflect their experience in precise language. Those who have never been ill might think that she is simply an agony aunt for the sick and that this book is a prototype for the self help genre. But they have never walked in this 'other country' of chronic sickness. Those who know well the experience can testify that what she says is absolutely true to the experience, as well as grounded in the Bible. It is written from a real place, because the 'reality' of the sick is reality, too. As she says in her book "You must always think of sickness as a hidden state, fully known only to its wayfarers".

Priscilla Maurice's theme is that chronic illness is a tool not to be despised, but to be accepted as something from God, to refine us. We must labour to get the goodness and growth out of it, as well as to try to recover from it. She is not

---
[1] From the Chapter "Days" (page 80)

against praying earnestly for healing even after many years of illness. She is against concentrating so much on being healed that we miss the deep sanctification that God is trying to develop in us.

She teaches us to take all things, including illness, as an essential part of Providence as if from God, and to co-operate with the bad things and not to fight against them. For Maurice, bad things are a kind of carefully measured vaccination, which, when properly administered and reacted to with faith, helps the body and mind to develop maturity and strength, which can be developed in no other way.

Priscilla Maurice also wished to better train those professionals who ministered to the sick. This book, carefully studied, offers useful approaches, if one has the insight and humility to listen carefully to what someone who has been ill, actually experiences. It may interest pastors and chaplains who want to understand better the more profound side of chronic illness and disability.

This message seems particularly urgent today since traditional Christian doctrine has been marginalised by humanistic teachings. This book bring us back to the 'basics' of faith, stripped of secondary worldly issues and to our duty to exercise critical self-analysis.

Priscilla Maurice wrote from a biblical point of view, drawing on hundreds of Scriptural texts, on Christian poetry and also on the original 'Service for the Visitation of the Sick'. As this is no longer familiar today, it is included in its original language at the end of this edition.

On almost all Victorian doctrinal debate, the author is silent. She is not distracted from the Bible's teaching. One can place her within the traditional Church of England without attempting to pin down her precise churchmanship. My conviction is that she would have described herself as a committed believer in the Thirty Nine Articles and the basic doctrines of the Reformation.

Sickness: its Trials and Blessings

When I first read Priscilla's book, I was myself struggling with a disbelieved, shattering, hidden and misunderstood chronic illness. Apart from the Psalms, the mysterious Book of Job, and nearly a thousand Bible texts on suffering, I found very little in modern church teaching or theology to describe the chronic malaise and bodily weakness I was suffering. I was aware that in this age of instant painkillers and anaesthetics, Christians must work hard to create a space for 'incurables'.

My experience of the Christian life did not fit in with the version of faith taught in many churches, which tends, either through fear of suffering to ignore, and therefore marginalise chronically sick members, or to recommend 'miraculous' healing, which in some cases, could be pretended, or even a short-lived delusion. God uses a diversity of ways to heal people, most commonly medical intervention. It is irresponsible to suggest to the sick, as Job's comforters did, that they may be ill *because* they do not believe enough in the Bible's healing promises. Some churches misapply Bible texts on healing. This book firmly contradicts all these approaches to chronic sickness, by making it clear that God can allow us to be ill for a greater reason.

In my experience, the chronically ill tend to accept the inevitable contradictions of actual life because they sense that to become whole, one needs real food, not 'fast food'. The Cross demonstrates that God uses suffering as the path to glory. There is short phase summing it all up: 'No pain, no gain'. Through coming to terms with frailty, we lay down all our weapons against God and we are healed of our deepest sickness, our hidden rebellion against Him. Then, He may graciously then deliver the spiritual growth and countless blessings from illness and disability, which are set out in this book and in the Bible.

I was so relieved when, as a newly confirmed Christian, I found this dusty, battered Victorian book and realized that my extreme experience of marginalization was shared by someone who had lived more than a century before me. Apart from anything else, I found in it a unique description of the world of chronic illness, from the inside. This gifted woman had walked through a similar wilderness and had been intellectually better prepared than me, to map it out.

I also knew that the author's quaint language was a barrier keeping this best-selling book from a wider, modern readership. I determined that if I ever recovered from my own chronic illness, I would publish the book under her name. I was, indeed, graciously healed after ten years, by a diversity of means. Some years of occasional reading in the British Library followed, which enabled me to pull together Priscilla Maurice's short biography. It took me two more years on and off, to render her words in contemporary English.

With the support of my husband, Paolo Castellina, an ordained minister and theologian, who has added some doctrinal footnotes, I have finally been been able to publish this modern version. Now, my chronically ill friends can fully meditate on Priscilla Maurice's work, liberated from their Victorian culture and phraseology. It is such a great comfort in illness to be offered systematic ideas that in one's general mental and physical weakness, one cannot pull together. Millions of people have endured chronic illness who have not had the intellectual capacity, stamina, strength and wisdom to write about it. This book does much of the work for them.

A friend once observed to me that that our shared chronic illness could contribute to a 'new spirituality'. What she really meant was that our contemporaries would return through suffering to the 'real food' of the truths of traditional Christianity. Traditional Christianity has been been suppressed by modern versions of Christianity, which, like humanistic teaching, prove inadequate in times of real testing, like chronic illness. Traditional Christian truth, firmly based on a complete understanding of the entire Bible, needs to be restored to the core of Western mainstream theology, for the sake of the sick, marginalized, disabled and suffering, even if no one else seems to desire it.

We hope that seekers after the truth will recognise that Priscilla Maurice's book is a spiritual classic, a rare description of that "wholly different state" of illness. How few people today analyse themselves, as the author did, to locate wrong thinking and to universalise their experience in the light of Scripture. In great weariness of body, soul and mind and without the use of a computer, this is her achievement. It remains impressive. Her mastery of Bible texts would be a feat for someone in perfect health, even today. Thus, we think that this book deserves to be an enduring Christian classic. We hope it will remain in print from now on, for the sake of those with chronic illnesses and disabilities.

In my view, Priscilla Maurice was a great woman and a great Christian. If we have been able to preserve and to share her work with a wider audience, in the spirit of her original mission, we will be very satisfied.

Alison Bailey Castellina M.A

London, June 2009

Editorial Technique

It has been my editorial policy to remove all linguistic obstacles by modernising the text, without radically altering the overall tone, style and meaning.

As an editor, my main aim has been to convey author's insights in more modern English without entirely losing the flavour of her Victorian phrasing, which conveys her character, epoch and personality. Wherever possible, we have made no changes at all but when necessary we have:

Sickness: its Trials and Blessings

a) broken up long sentences and paragraphs, to support readers with chronic illness, in their reading;

b) made slight alterations to the author's phraseology, without changing its meaning and emotional power. For example "by degrees" is not always but often rendered by "gradually", "shall" is often changed to "will", commas are removed before "and" and there are obsolete words and phrases like "shrink from" and "repine" that have to be replaced. Victorian spellings (which were like modern American ones) e.g. endings -or have been replaced with –our;

c) sometimes rendered the word "sickness" by "illness", "tried" by "tested" but have left the words "sickness" and "trials" in the title;

d) modified outmoded medical treatments. For example, we have altered the chapter entitled "Opiates" to "Drugs" but have inserted a note about the use of opiates;

e) modified old fashioned ways of life and customs, such as the author's assumption that the reader will have their own servant. This can be distracting when reading the text;

f) updated references to noise from horses and carriages in the street to the noise of modern traffic;

g) added some modern diseases like AIDS to her lists of conditions and inserted "communications" for letters e.g. meaning phone or email;

h) modernised the biblical references.

Where we have discovered the course of a quotation or have a comment in relation to the text, we have inserted footnotes and cross references.

All Priscilla Maurice's original footnotes are now embedded in the text as Bible quotations.

A Gift to the Sick

As Job says "*When He has tested me I shall come forth as gold*". We hope that those who read this book will come to love and to cherish it. We hope to publish a free study guide (on http://fatigue.wikispaces.com) to help people to make it their own. Some may wish to give it those who are chronically or terminally ill. It could be used for sermon source material or offer insights to those who minister to the sick and dying, such as chaplains and pastors.

Other books by Priscilla Maurice:

- Help and Comfort for the Sick Poor (published 1853)
- Prayers for the Sick and Dying (published 1853)
- Sacred Poems for Mourners (published 1846)

Dedications

We are dedicating this updated version of the book to the memory of Priscilla Maurice, Emma Maurice; Deanne and to the memory of Olwyn Moore, who admired Priscilla Maurice's writing, during her own last illness.

Alison Bailey Castellina M.A

Paolo Castellina B.D

London, June 2009

Sickness: its Trials and Blessings

Biographical Note on Priscilla Maurice

Priscilla Maurice was born into one of the most gifted families of Victorian Britain. The Maurice family was earnest, brilliant and influential. They mixed with people like Gladstone, Tennyson, Thomas Carlyle, Charles Kingsley and Edward Strachey. Maurice men and women notably had a seriousness of mind which we hardly understand today. For example, the Maurice women wrote theological letters to one another while living under the same roof. No doubt, this honed their writing skills.

Priscilla Maurice's own writing style has authority, lyricism, sensitivity and compassion. She is not just a product of the superficially pious Victorian age, but she added to that, her own particularly deep understanding of human psychology. In addition, to her written skills, Priscilla Maurice was highly gifted at comforting others. Her primary desire in life was to go overseas as a missionary, but she instead she became a kind of missionary to the sick, in England.

Priscilla Hurrey Maurice (1811-1854) was born in Normanton, Suffolk, one of the youngest children of Michael Maurice, a Unitarian Minister, founder of The Unitarian Society and of Priscilla Hurrey, daughter of a Great Yarmouth timber merchant. Michael met his wife through teaching her Classics.

Priscilla had elder sisters, Elizabeth Mary and Anne who were nearly fifteen years older than a cluster of younger sisters and their famous brother, John Frederick Denison[2] (1805-1872). He was known to twentieth century admirers, such as Archbishop of Canterbury Michael Ramsay as 'F. D. Maurice'. Among the younger Maurice sisters, Priscilla had an elder sister Emma (born 1807) and younger twin sisters Jane and Lucilla (born 1814). Her youngest sisters were the

---
[2]Details on John Denison Maurice from "The Dictionary of National Biography"

future wife of the Dean of Wells, Harriet Theodosia and Esther, future wife of Julius Hare, a don at Trinity College Cambridge.

In 1812, the large Maurice family moved to Clifton and then in 1813, they moved to Frenchay near Bristol, where the Unitarian Chapel, built in 1685 still stands. Under the influence of their Hurrey cousins who stayed with them until their deaths in the winter of 1814-15, her elder sisters read the Bible for themselves and were convinced that it did not teach their father's Unitarianism which was 'one God' but the Trinity of Father, Son and Holy Spirit.

Being strong individuals, like most of the Maurice family, the elder sisters, aged nearly 20, refused to continue to attend the Unitarian Chapel. A family 'crisis' followed as their mother also refused to attend. The content of their mother's letter telling her husband that she could no longer be a Unitarian still exists. Instead of Unitarianism, the individualistic Maurice women eventually took up with no single denomination. Elizabeth (born 1795) became Anglican and Anne (born 1977) became a Baptist with a strong Calvinist flavour. Mary (born 1796) became a Methodist.

Possibly under the influence of her eldest sister Elizabeth, Priscilla Maurice, who was sixteen years her junior, became, in essence, a devout Anglican, with a Calvinist streak. French-born Jean Calvin (1509 - 1564) was a prominent advocate of the five 'solas' of the Reformation ("by grace alone, by the authority of Scripture alone, by faith alone, through Christ alone, for the glory of God"). He taught that the Bible alone and not church tradition and leadership, is the final authority for all matters of faith and that salvation itself is attained purely through free grace without any contribution from the good works of the believer. Calvin is also widely known for his teaching on absolute predestination and election, often regarded as determinism, though Calvin himself, and his followers, strongly rejected this, and argued for personal responsibility.

Calvin taught that the saved, the 'elect' (a word that Priscilla once uses) are those for whom Christ died on the Cross[3]. Thus, Calvinism was too narrow for more liberal Victorian universalism which held that all men are saved[4]. Predestination in Calvinism was a sticking point for many in a faith that was otherwise regarded as having great purity and clarity.

Calvinism has produced two great English writers, John Bunyan and Charles Haddon Spurgeon. Calvinism's characteristic systematic approach is also reflected in the inspired way that Priscilla Maurice catalogues aspects of what is otherwise the almost indefinable experience of chronic sickness. Calvinism also encourages believers to do everything to the glory of God. This could be the reason why the author remained anonymous in her published work. Jean Calvin himself did not allow his name to appear on his own tombstone. The author, too, would do everything for the glory of God, and not for personal fame.

Young Priscilla was taught, together with F. D. Maurice[5] and her sister Emma, by a Unitarian governess. F .D. Maurice went on to attend Trinity College Cambridge and took a first class honours degree in law, though later became Professor of English Literature at London University. He shared a deep love of English literature with Priscilla, who particularly loved the English Christian poets, Henry Vaughan and

---

[3] This is the doctrine of limited atonement, one of the five points of Reformed theology. They are: total depravity, unconditional election, limited atonement, irresistible grace and perseverance of the saints. Refer: http://en.wikipedia.org/wiki/Calvinism

[4] F. D. Maurice was "misty" on this doctrine. He was not a "universalist" but he qualified a belief in election by asserting that for some unbelievers there will be some kind of salvation. He was not accepted as "orthodox" by evangelicals.

[5] The Life of Frederick Denison Maurice (Chiefly in his own Letters). Edited by his son, Sir Frederick Maurice (published 1884).

George Herbert and, judging by unattributed quotations in this book, the poems of John Keble in 'The Christian Year'.

F.D. Maurice and his sisters had strong literary leanings. His first book was a novel 'Eustace Conway'. Priscilla's first publication was extracts of great English poetry about death ('Sacred Poems for Mourners'). Clearly, they were both highly responsive to the English language. F.D Maurice founded magazines at University and contributed to the Athenaeum and Westminster Review magazines.

Young Priscilla, like many young gifted Victorian women, had to endure harsh educational and social restraints. She also had to bear a string of shattering bereavements, which must have cast her, at an early age, upon faith and on the hope of seeing loved ones again. First, there were the untimely deaths of both her inspiring Hurrey cousins who had been used in the Christian conversions within the family. Then, the eldest sister, Elizabeth became an invalid and brought up the twins, Jane and Anne, in her sick room. Then, in June 1831, in Southampton, where the Maurice family moved in 1827, Priscilla's beloved elder sister Emma fell mortally ill, at the age of twenty four, when Priscilla was just twenty. This sad event in some ways shaped the course of the entire Maurice family history. The manner of Emma's death made a deep impression, not only on Priscilla but also on her brother who, until Emma's illness had been interested in philosophy and literature. After this, he accepted the Thirty-Nine Articles of the Anglican Church, and Priscilla felt called to become a missionary. F. D. Maurice soon took Anglican Holy Orders, studying alongside Gladstone at Exeter College, Oxford.

At home, in 1831, in Southampton for his summer break, F. D. Maurice stayed close to dying Emma during her last weeks. Unlike her other sisters, who were more forceful and individualistic, Emma seems to have been one of those sweet, gentle souls, possibly like Beth in "Little Women".

Sickness: its Trials and Blessings

The extent to which her death affected them both is evident in the fact that in July 1851, F. D. Maurice joined Priscilla on the twentieth anniversary of Emma's death to remember her. Brother and sister also had to endure the deaths of their younger twins, Jane and Lucilla. Out of the original extended family of ten children, including their Hurrey first cousins, they lost five to an early death, through illness.

Priscilla's call to become an overseas missionary never came to fruition. She later said that she felt that God put obstacles in her way. From about the time of her sister's death in 1831 until about 1836, she fulfilled the role of her brother's housekeeper. It is clear that her health was reasonably robust. During this period, two of her sisters married. Harriet Maurice married into the Dean of Wells and Esther Maurice married the Cambridge don, Julius Hare, who was also an ordained minister. Mary worked as a governess.

Portraits of her brother, F. D. Maurice show a refined, kind and sensitive face. Revd. Charles Kingsley thought Maurice was "the most beautiful human soul" he had ever met. Others thought him "saintlike". Priscilla Maurice may have had a similar face. However, we cannot tell, as no portraits of her have so far emerged. Alfred, Lord Tennyson thought F. D. Maurice was one of the greatest minds of the Victorian age and would not hear a word against him. A most balanced view comes from Benjamin Jowett[6] who, possibly more perceptively, said that,

"Maurice was misty and confused. But he was a great man and a disinterested nature and he always stood by anyone who appeared to be oppressed".

His gifted sister, Priscilla, also had a great mind. She was also blessed with a gift of extraordinary clarity and psychological insight. Even in illness, she could think clearly both

---

[6]The Life and Letters of Benjamin Jowett : E Abbott and L Campbell (published 1897).

about human psychology and Scripture, which is a great feat.

With so many gifted sisters, F. D. Maurice was clearly an admirer of the female intellect. He was close to the movers of the suffragette movement and to intellectual Christian women like Dorothea Beale, the founder of St Hilda's College, Oxford. He founded an establishment in Harley Street for the higher education of women, which became Queen's College, London University. He was a key champion of the women's university movement. No doubt, he justly sensed that it was completely unacceptable that women, such as his sisters were deprived of degrees and careers, which their male counterparts freely enjoyed.

From 1835-1846, F .D. Maurice was the chaplain at Guy's Hospital, London. His mother and Priscilla ran his household before he married, and after he married they continued to live with him. The census of March 1841 shows that F. D. Maurice was living within Guy's Hospital with his wife Ann (Barton) and their son. Priscilla, Jane and their mother were living with him. There can be little doubt that Priscilla would either have met, or heard a lot about her brother's friends, Carlyle, Kingsley, Gladstone and Tennyson.

Priscilla, deprived of a higher education and profession, seems to have been dependent on her brother. By the late 1840s, she was the last of the Calvinist Anglicans in the family. Before she was ill, she could get out to church and mix easily with similar minds. But there must have been the constant worry about her finances and this, as well as so much bereavement in her life, which can damage immunity, could have undermined her general health. For me, it is not surprising that sometime in the 1840s, Priscilla fell chronically ill with what seems to have been regarded only a nervous condition, but which was probably an organic and physical condition about which little was understood. It seems to me that part of her condition involved severe digestive problems. Without doubt, her illness was extremely debilitating.

It seems to me that Priscilla Maurice may well have ministered unofficially at Guy's visiting sick patients. This would have alleviated some of the workload of her brother who was busy preparing to take up the post of Professor of History and English Literature at Kings College, London, as well as writing his many books and articles. Certainly, she seems to have had a very wide experience of illness and death beds, drawn from the sick rooms of Elizabeth and Emma, but also from her time at Guy's Hospital, London.

Tragically, in 1845, F. D. Maurice's first wife, Ann Barton died, leaving two young sons. It was in that year that Priscilla Maurice published her first book 'Sacred Poems for Mourners', a moving and inspirational collection of poems on death by Herbert, Vaughan, Milton and lesser known contemporary poets. This reflects her habitual reading of Christian poetry which is apparent in this book in her short unattributed quotations in verse. The publication of her first book in 1845 may have been in response to another death in the Maurice family, as well in response to her sense that she should try to earn her living through writing. Surrounded by death, she was starting to think deeply about the meaning of suffering and to glean insights from the literary treasury of Christian poetry, itself inspired by Scripture.

The death of Ann Maurice could have profoundly shaken F. D. Maurice's faith. But he was secure in that at least, and he married, in 1849, Georgiana Hare-Naylor, sister-in-law of Julius Hare of Herstmonceux Castle. At this point, it is possible that Priscilla moved to Hastings. In 1853, F. D. Maurice who refused to join any church 'party' and did not believe strictly in eternal punishment was effectively dismissed from his post at King's College, London, for publishing a book regarded as unorthodox. Living by now in Russell Square, he founded the Working Men's Colleges. Later, in 1860, in spite

Sickness: its Trials and Blessings

of objections from twenty two evangelical clergymen, F. D. Maurice was appointed Priest-in-Charge at The Oxford Chapel or St Peter's Church, Vere Street, now part of All Souls Church, Langham Place. Tennyson and Gladstone, needless to say, supported his appointment and, at least, he gained a living there.

A visit to Priscilla's sick room in Hastings in 1854 is recorded by her nephew, the travel writer Augustus Hare, in Chapter VI of his biography "The Story of my Life[7]" in which is noted that family members knelt, while taking Communion by her bed.

Priscilla Maurice left London for the salt air of Hastings, to live at White Rock Place, 10, Caroline Place, St Mary in Castle, Hastings. She seems to have lived in three rooms in a house which took gentlewomen lodgers. The area was, at that time, full of elegant, terraced, lodging houses for well-to-do women with a need for the reviving seaside. Priscilla had a small legacy or annuity and regularly had guests to stay. Augustus Hare tells us that her bedroom had wide views of the Channel, since Caroline Place, now demolished, was directly on the seafront. After years of being confined in viewless rooms in London, Priscilla enjoyed the sea views from her upstairs windows.

The census (1851) records the author as the head of the household, living alone with one servant, Eliza Perkins as an 'annuitant' (living on an annuity). It also records that she had a visitor, her friend Caroline from Putney. We can imagine that in Hastings, she had a regular stream of visitors, including her brother. There is a hint in one of his letters that she was able, at one point, to go on a local sea cruise.

As a communicant of the Church of England, Priscilla was acquainted with the vicar of St Leonards on Sea, near Hastings, Revd F C Massingberd. It seems that she asked him to write a short introduction to her work 'Sickness: Its Trials

---

[7] See http://augustus-hare.tripod.com

Sickness: its Trials and Blessings

and Blessings'. The book was an immediate success reprinted seven times over the next thirty years.

Priscilla's book is a kind of exploration of the Order of the Visitation of the Sick, which was part of the Book of Common Prayer. In the same way, her book 'Sacred Poems for Mourners' explores the Burial Service. Whether consciously or not, her writing supplements F. D. Maurice's own writing on the Book of Common Prayer.

The Maurice sisters' differing doctrines may have put pressure on their brother to seek a bastion against the various strands of Protestant Christian doctrine in his own family. F. D. Maurice wrote this about the Book of Common Prayer: *"The Book of Common Prayer is my protection and the protection of the Church against Anglicanism and Evangelicalism and Liberalism and Romanism and Rationalism and, until these different devils cease to torment me, I will with God's help, use this shield against them"* (Life of F. D. Maurice, Letters).

The Maurice family's social circles had brought Priscilla into direct contact with leading clergymen. Judging from comments in this book, it could have her sense of disappointment at how Anglican clergy approached her own long illness that motivated her to write this book. Clearly, from the evidence of a letter to her, F. D. Maurice did not feel he could minister to her, in spite of having been Chaplain at Guy's Hospital, a role for which, he said, he was "entirely inadequate". If the majority of Victorian clergy felt inadequate in relation to the chronically sick, it is not surprising that "Sickness Its Trials and Blessings" was reprinted so many times, from 1850 onwards.

In 1853, Priscilla Maurice published another two books, *'Help and Comfort for the Sick Poor'* which is a shilling version of *'Sickness: its Trials and Blessings'* with some added material. By 1853, her style is more confident. She is more at peace and less mentally frail. She knew she would leave her mark. She knew by this time, that her specialist ministry to the sick was widely appreciated. In 1853, she also published *'Prayers for the Sick and Dying'*. It does not seem that in 1850 when she wrote *'Sickness: its Trials and Blessings'* that she thought she was dying, but by 1853, she may have suspected it. She died the following year in June 1854, at the age of 43, in Hastings.

After being appointed Professor of Moral Theology and Philosophy at Cambridge, F. D. Maurice died in 1872. He was buried in the Maurice family vault, in a corner of Highgate Cemetery although many had wanted him to bury him in Westminster Abbey.

The circles in which Priscilla Maurice moved were dominated by well-educated, lively and spiritually-minded women and energetic, scholarly Christian reformers, often decades ahead of their time. F. D. Maurice's efforts bore secular fruit, in the 20th century's championing of women's higher education and in the concept of "Christian Socialism" both of which have profoundly shaped the modern world. His message is worth considering today, for Maurice was against both 'unsocial Christianity' and 'unchristian Socialism'. But he, unlike Priscilla Maurice, tried to sit on the fence over the authority of the Bible. For Priscilla Maurice, Scripture remained the only authority. It is Priscilla Maurice's strong biblical faith that enabled her to tackle with power and understanding, extreme human experiences. Her mental achievement, while seriously ill, in applying hundreds of biblical texts to illness, is one reason why the book is still relevant.

Her main theme is that every aspect of suffering is in the hands of an all loving God, who uses every aspect of every situation to develop and discipline those whom He loves to make them more like His Son. She applies this to every circumstance, often with great creativity.

Sickness: its Trials and Blessings

At times, in spite of one's admiration for her, one wonders how much Priscilla Maurice was an exacting spirit. She was, evidently full of warmth and compassion for those suffering, but there are a few indications that she may also have been a little relentless in her pursuits and had to master impatience, when interrupted. She might have been, unintentionally, a little intimidating.

Nor did she pretend to virtues that have not been developed in the fiery furnace. There is a sense in her writing of sin taken seriously, reminiscent of John Bunyan. Priscilla's other theme is to encourage others to see their own illness as a visitation from God, even a kind of special privilege for Christian 'soldiers'.

Unlike F. D. Maurice, Priscilla's faith was traditional and, in that sense, her ideas have transcended the passing of time. In fact, her brother's lofty but 'misty' topics seem comparatively irrelevant today, even if his influence continues in secular liberalism. F. D. Maurice's glittering worldly achievements make one wonder what Priscilla Maurice saw as the meaning of her own limited life. For me, it is clear that in spite of living under his shadow, Priscilla Maurice strongly believed that through her writing, she had a serious and mysterious secret calling, which was to minister comfort to people whom she would never know in her earthly life.

Both F. D. Maurice and Priscilla Maurice were great Victorians. Both were brilliant, high minded, passionate, caring and literary people. They both attempted to lighten the path of those suffering and to bring real hope and comfort. Both left behind them enduring works. But for me, it was Priscilla Maurice, the vulnerable but strong minded woman, who loved the Bible who was the greater of the two.

Sadly, F. D. Maurice was prevented from writing a preface to his sister's book, which was published anonymously by his own publisher Rivingtons. It is interesting to note that F. D. Maurice's descendants were also writers, as well as distinguished generals and Cambridge academics. Literature and academic achievements continues to run strongly in the Maurice line.

Writing is one thing, but service to mankind is another. Amazingly, Priscilla Maurice, who had almost no strength and only very limited means, achieved ongoing work for those in need. Our research demonstrates that Priscilla provided in her will for a convalescent care home for sick women, in Hastings. She may have used money from the sale of this book which continued to be a best-seller until the end of the 19th century. Between 1855 and 1902, nurses and medical professionals cared for almost two thousand women in her 'Home for Invalided Gentlewomen' ('Catherine House') St Leonards-on-Sea, which was purpose-built in 1862. It was designed as a 'refined' comfortable home for the temporary care of invalided ladies with very limited means. By 1902, it could house 22 sick women in eleven bedrooms[8] and needed to appeal for donations in 'The Times'.

In another religious tradition, Priscilla Maurice might be considered a saint. But Protestants firmly reject saints, knowing that all achievements rest upon divine 'grace'. It is our pleasure, therefore, in this modernised version to add Priscilla Maurice's authorship to the title of her book and to tell her inspiring story. It is our hope that her wholehearted blessing would have rested upon our endeavours to introduce to a wider audience this book, which was written for the glory of God.

---

[8]From a description of Catherine House in The Times, 2 January 1902

Preface by a Minister of Religion (1850)

The author of this book has herself been tested by long years of sickness and has asked a friend to certify his belief, as a clergyman, that this book is not inconsistent with the teaching of the Church of England, with Scripture, the fountain of true consolation and with showing how to apply them. It was a careful study of The Service for the Visitation of the Sick that first taught her the meaning and the blessings of sickness. Her desire has been that it may be instrumental in pointing out to others the same sources of consolation.

It is not intended that every part of this book should apply to every case but it is hoped that something may be gained by many sufferers, in a variety of conditions, from the experiences of someone who has passed through the stages of sickness. Comfort may be derived from the discovery that others sufferers have felt the same.

It is most often through suffering that the Lord's people are made like Him. They are "never so truly happy," as when they are learning in that which one of our martyred Reformers called "Christ's Own Sweet School."[9]

The name of a clergyman can give no authority and scarcely any recommendation to this book but it is added at the request of the author, in full agreement with all that she has written.

F. C. Massingberd

St. Leonards-on-Sea, March 20, 1850

---

[9] This quotation is reported as by Cranmer in the "Life of Archbishop Cranmer" by William Gilpin published by Rivingtons in 1819.

Sickness: its Trials and Blessings

Sickness: its Trials and Blessings

Part I - New Ways of Looking at Illness

Introduction

Each of us knows that we must die alone but how few of us realise that, for the most part, it is God's will that each one of us must live alone, and suffer alone?

Each of us "*will have to bear his own load*" (Galatians 6:5) and feel his own incommunicable pain which "often lies like lead upon the heart, or like ice within the heart"[10].

A deep sense of isolation is not unique to sickness. Those who are successful in the world have their own loneliness of heart and find it hard to bear. This deep, weary sense of isolation is a call to the sick to sympathise with and to better understand the trials of those who have health.

There is in every heart, a craving for sympathy and it is a restless craving in those who have never learned where to turn for true sympathy and that God is the "One only and only One" who is enough to satisfy all our needs.

There are few who do not feel pained that their problems and isolation are not better understood by others. They think they ought to be, they expect sympathy, they crave it. They cry *"out in their pain"* (Isaiah 26:17) that their lot is hard and peculiar and that life is not so bad for others. They go on complaining so loudly and so constantly that they do not, except occasionally hear *"the still, small voice"* which is speaking to them, and saying, *"Listen to me"*. When they do, it tells them that their lot is not unique or peculiar, but the lot common to Mankind.

Each one of us, in his or her own way, or rather in the way that God sees fitted to his character, is living alone. Some more so, some less so. There is a meaning in it all, an abso-

---
[10] This appears to be a quotation, but it is unattributed in the original.

lute necessity. Those who *"Hear of the rod and of him who appointed it"* (Micah 6:9) will then no longer feel isolated and will understand that the whole point of their suffering is to withdraw them from others, from themselves, from the cravings for materialism and passion and to drive them to find comfort and relief in God alone, and to live in Him.

The lesson is always the same. But there are different ways of learning it. The individual path which each man or woman walks is not trodden by any one else. From the outside, we cannot judge its unevenness, or how much pain there is in it.

No one can fully see the extent and details of the suffering which someone else is bearing. One person speaks words of sympathy for one part of a trial, another for some other part. A third sees no trial at all and a fourth thinks it must be much less difficult to bear than some other form of suffering, or than his or her own. No one except the sufferer sees all its inward suffering. No one else can feel your own acute pain.

So each comforter leaves disappointment behind or else makes the sufferer think, "I would be entirely without comfort (or at least only very imperfectly understood) if I had my fellow-sufferers only to depend on. Each sufferer seems wrapped in his or her own sorrow with eyes too intently fixed on it to see my suffering, except dimly". They must appeal to Him who "weighs the spirits".

The weight of life is difficult to bear, at the best of times. How much more so, when there is sickness, as well. Then, there is added the weary longing to make a contribution and to live. But there are empty days which all seem devoted to 'self' and in which one never seems to do anything for others, except to add to their burdens.

One can become depressed as time passes and brings no relief. Each morning seems just to begin another day of selfishness. You feel you could do something, but what you can't decide what, nor where to turn for occupation.

Your friends may know you are not well enough to work and in kindness, or so they think, remove jobs from you. They tell you that you are not needed, that there are plenty of others who can take your place. They mean this kindly, but you do not feel it as kindness. If you could only find a niche and be useful again, you would be so thankful. Not being useful in the world is part of the burden. Remember too, that you cannot truly feel the love that makes your friends speak as they do.

Be patient and wait. Don't rebel but instead just lie still. Don't say, "I am cut off from life and work and so there is nothing left for me, no point in living". Things may change. Don't lose the blessing of your present state in reaching after something either, future or imaginary. Look for what your work is now. Don't ask to have your world enlarged but just to fulfil your present role which is to find your present ministry.

For example, you could be a blessing to your carer. If your carer sees you patient and submissive in your situation, bearing pain patiently, receiving life cheerfully and not complaining about the illness or about God, he or she may learn a lesson which may sink deep into their heart and produce future spiritual fruit.

You may have a ministry to your family. Do you have parents, or brothers, or sisters, or children living under the same roof with you? Merely talking to them cheerfully, making them feel that they are always welcome, that you are ever ready to share their problems, sympathising with them, sharing their interests and pleasures as well as their sorrows will make your illness a blessing for them. Your house may become blessed for your sake because God who has linked you to the "prisoners and captives" can bless you, and *"the places all around my hill"* (Ezekiel 34:26).

Sickness: its Trials and Blessings

In this over-active world, many are looking for some place of refreshment where they can leave behind them the jarring of life and draw nearer to reality. Don't say in your heart that that you have no job. Instead, lie back and let Him *"who works in you, both to will and to work for his good pleasure"* (Philippians 2:13). Ask Jesus to make you so like Himself that others may take note that you *"have been with Jesus"* (Acts 4:13). Continually refresh yourself in Him and then water others, *"so that we may be able to comfort those who are in any affliction, with the comfort with which we ourselves are comforted by God."* (2 Corinthians 1:4)

You have a great work to do. It is to say 'No' to *"ungodliness and worldly passion"* (Timothy 2:12) and *"to walk humbly with your God"* (Micah 6:8). This ministry is glorious and honourable. So don't despise it in case you *"complain against God"* (Romans 9:20) and tempt Him to withdraw the test. Besides, even if it were true that you have nothing to do, no outward life, you have one stone in His Temple to polish. That stone is yourself and this time of illness is given to you to do this.

Consider it as a time of preparation, although you do not know what for. It may be for life, or it may be for death. But do not waste time. Don't waste it by complaining or crying out for some alteration. God sees your heart and knows that this test is hard and He is *"compassionate and merciful"* (James 5:11). He sees that you need precisely this discipline and He will give you no other discipline until this test has done the work for which He sent it.

At this very moment, many others are suffering, in mind and body, just as you are suffering. They have the same problems, pains and temptations even though you don't know them and they know nothing of you. Nor are you ever likely to meet until the day when *"the purposes of the heart"* are disclosed (1 Corinthians 4:5).

Sickness: its Trials and Blessings

How you suffer is very important to them because, unknown to you, you affect them, even though you do not indeed exactly know how. Every member of the Body of Christ is necessary to, and affects the whole Body. A realisation of this truth will not only take away the loneliness of sickness but will also prevent the feeling of your life being useless and sickness being meant only for an individual's increase in personal holiness.

The Creed says, "I believe in the communion of Saints" and so I am not alone. I cannot be alone because my trial is not mine alone. My conflicts and my temptations are those of some other member of Christ's Church. In fighting them, I fight for them, as well as for myself. In overcoming temptations or unbelief, I weaken Satan's power over them, as well as over myself.

"No temptation has overtaken you that is not common to man" (1 Corinthians 10:13). Surely no one sick should ever say, "Mine is the hardest suffering, the most difficult form of suffering". How can you know unless you have tasted them all?[11] Even if it is the hardest, then it is the most blessed for you and the most helpful for sick and suffering fellow believers.

These ideas, truly internalised, would gradually remove your feeling of isolation which is so common and so painful in long illness.

Who hath the Father and the Son,

---

[11] Christ bore for us the hardest suffering: *"He was despised and rejected by men; a man of sorrows, and acquainted with grief; and as one from whom men hide their faces; he was despised, and we esteemed him not. Surely he has borne our griefs and carried our sorrows; yet we esteemed him stricken, smitten by God, and afflicted. But he was wounded for our transgressions; he was crushed for our iniquities; upon him was the chastisement that brought us peace, and with his stripes we are healed. All we like sheep have gone astray; we have turned—every one—to his own way; and the Lord has laid on him the iniquity of us all"* (Isaiah 53:3-6).

May be left, but not alone[12].

1.1 First Impressions of a Long Illness or Chronic Condition

So an illness has come upon you. Have you just started to realise that you cannot hope that it will simply disappear and that it is even likely to be a lifelong condition? Suddenly you are depressed. You feel *"your whole heart faint"* (Isaiah 1:5) and that you are in *"the land of gloom like thick darkness, like deep shadow without any order, where light is as thick darkness."* (Job 10:22).

Actually, when an illness starts, it does not seem so dark. God deals with us gently. He does not let us see the future length of the illness ahead. He hides its full length, in case we should give up or lose heart. He gives us comforts to the extent that He makes make things pleasant what would otherwise be unbearable.

At first, God showers upon us the kindness of friends, their sympathy, their nurturing care and concern. It seems as if the world is centred on us, as if we were the only focus of life. All this is very pleasant. All our desires are anticipated, almost before we had expressed them. We seem to understand that our friends have a deep concern and love for us, that we never knew before. We feel that we have value and importance for them in a way that we had never dreamed of and that their very happiness hangs upon our well-being. They seem to live in and through us.

It is well worth the counterbalance of a great deal of distress and suffering to experience such love. We seem introduced into a new world where there is only love, kindness, consideration and sympathy and from which all the anxieties and

---
[12]This quotation is taken from "St John's Day" a poem in "The Christan Year" (for Sunday and Holidays) compiled by Revd John Keble published in 1827.

Sickness: its Trials and Blessings

frustrations of life are excluded. The reason for this is that our friends have pity on us.

So what do we know, at this point, of the 'test of faith'? We never had such attention and love before. Why? Because it is all gathered up into a brief space. But the time is coming when love and tenderness may no longer be shown. Quite soon, the first crisis of the illness subsides and for a while, there is relief and joy because you seem to be returning to health. But God has appointed otherwise. It is not His Will to give you health, but a long-drawn out, possibly even a life-long, chronic condition.

Now, for the first time, you start to become aware of the real 'test'. At first, when the novelty of the state has passed away and a changed, narrowed prospect lies before you, it seems full of sorrow, as if it will never end.

Years of suffering? How the mind recoils at such a thought! Is there no prospect of some gradual recovery? No, the opposite may be true. The condition may get worse. It is useless to say, *"I loathe my life"* (Job 10:1) and *"so that I prefer strangling and death, rather than this body of mine"* (Job 7:15,16 NIV). This is not the answer. This will not lighten the heavy burden which you feel too heavy to be borne. Don't say, *"Hold your peace with me, and let me speak, then let come on me what may!"* (Job 13:13 NKJV)". Don't say *"It is hopeless"* (Isaiah 57:10) for it is not. Your present state is one full of tests, temptations, depression, distress and insecurity. But you must believe, equally, that it is full of blessings, full of comforts, mercies, work and enjoyments too. Believe this is true, even though now it seems to you that this advice is like "one who mocks".

Apply your heart to the Word of God *"Apply your heart to instruction and your ear to words of knowledge"* (Proverbs 23:12), and the time will not be far distant when you will see the "rainbow in the clouds" and learn who put it there and see each day a "rainbow in every storm".

At the moment, you cannot "*look on the light when it is bright in the skies when the wind has passed and cleared them*" (Job 37:21). But it will one day be *"like the light when it is bright in the skies, when the wind has passed and cleared them ... like the sun shining forth on a cloudless morning"* (2 Samuel 23:4). What if the rains come first?

Don't be afraid for the flood will not drown you, because the Lord will be with you. You must try to focus on the good things and blessings which issue from illness, separately from its hardships. This cannot be simply done because the blessings are so inextricably connected with the hardships. You often think that the pain in itself would not be hard to bear but that the torture is in its interference, as you see it, with your life's work and its inconvenience for others.

Be assured that this illness does not interfere with your life's work and calling. What God calls you to, He will give you strength for. You do not have the inner strength previously, or in yourself, but if He calls you to something, He will give the measure of strength required at the time, and for that particular thing.

The illness seems to interfere with the lives of other people. But they need the trial of your sickness, as much as you do. It will, in its way be as much a blessing for them as for you. Leave it all to God. *"Commit your way to the LORD; trust in him, and he will act"* (Psalms 37:5).

1.2 Illness: A Hidden State

The longer an illness continues, the more you learn that illness is a hidden state. Much of that portion of your life, which in health would be seen and shared by others, is now hidden from their eyes, from all eyes, except those of *"your Father who sees in secret"* (Matthew 9:24). You will now have to learn that few people understand your state at all and that even those who really want to, make great mistakes, which often gives you great and, you tend to think, needless pain.

If you bear in mind your own previous ignorance of the state of illness, how day by day, hidden things are revealed to you too, you will be less surprised that others do not know the lengths, breadths, depths and heights of your distress.

Each person must pass through illness to know the way and to be enabled to point out the road and its turnings and landmarks to others. Beware, therefore, of expecting too much and of taking it for granted that everyone sees and knows your pain and ought to avoid adding to it. Do not always be looking out for this kind of understanding. Do not expect to meet with it often. Then you will be spared much bitter disappointment and sorrow of heart. Doubtless, if some of your pains were seen and fully understood, your friends would try to remove them. But how many blessings would you lose? These little tests "reveal the thoughts of the heart". You cannot give them up and do not wish to get rid of them for *"he does not willingly afflict or grieve the children of men."* (Lamentations 3:33) He Himself would remove them unless He saw that they were *necessary* for you.

Try not to think, "These trifles which are too much for me and yet could be so easily removed. They do no good and they are too little to bring about anything positive. They only produce frustration and stir up sinful thoughts in me". Well, then, if they can produce so much evil, why can't they produce an equal measure of good? Their very trivial character makes them useful. They develop Christian character in you, secretly, insignificantly, and yet sharply. Think of the crown of thorns borne for you. Did that cause no suffering? Yet, what are thorns?

It is no use hiding from yourself that from now on you are going to be developed and tested. Face it all. Look fully at it and expect suffering. Receive it as your daily portion. When you say *"Give us this day our daily bread,"* (Matthew 6:11)

37

remember that you are asking for your daily portion of suffering. But never forget also that you are asking for your daily portion of strength, which you will also receive.

It is best to look upon illness as a state wholly different from any condition that you have ever yet known. It involves a wholly different set of distresses, temptations, trials and blessings. It is not to be looked at or treated like the state of health. Look upon each little struggle as a trial i.e. as meaning *"that he might humble you, testing you to know what was in your heart, whether you would keep his commandments or not."* (Deuteronomy 8:2)".

It is a painful thing to feel as if you are in a cage in illness and it offers the constant temptation to beat your wings against the sides of it. But stay on your perch quietly and you will not feel the bondage and imprisonment of your cage. After all, it is God who has shut you in and therefore you are safe there, and only there.

You must not expect that illness will ever become a pleasant thing, a condition without great pain and distress. But would you wish this to be the case? What blessing can you expect from any state, without pain? What could you learn from it? How would it liken you to your Master, who was made *"perfect through suffering"* (Hebrews 2:10)? *"For the Lord disciplines the one he loves, and chastises every son whom he receives"* (Hebrews 12:1).

Do you want to be deprived of this token of His esteem? You would do well to make up your mind not to expect or desire this. Face the whole trial. Don't draw back from acknowledging to yourself that illness is full of distress and testing and will always be so as long as it lasts. It is meant to be. As soon as you get used to any portion, it stops distressing you and then it stops blessing you. At that point, the God of Love will change it for some other form of discipline. *"He Himself went not up to joy, but first He suffered pain. He entered not into His glory before He was crucified"* (Hebrews 12.10).

So our way to eternal joy is to suffer here with Christ, and our door to enter into eternal life is gladly to die with Christ, that we may rise again from death and dwell with Him in everlasting life" (from The Service for The Visitation of the Sick).

1.3 The Twofold Character of Illness

If we consider our illness as our own private property which has reference only to ourselves it becomes just that: our own private property. Its lessons are personal and so are its blessings. Instead, we must never lose sight of the twofold character of our illness.

Illness is personal and meant for our individual profit, *"...that we may share his holiness"* (Hebrews 12:10). It is intended to make us more like Jesus, "to increase divine grace in you, to add strength to your faith and seriousness to your repentance" (Service for The Visitation of the Sick[13]) and to make repentance real, deep and earnest, as never before.

Illness is intended to mould your will to God's will, to dissolve you until you are lost in Him. It is to correct you and develop you, and for your chastening from past and present sins. It is to change the appearance of the earth and of your fellow human beings to show them in their true light, to show their inadequacies, in contrast to God.

Illness is intended to show what others can do in relation to your needs, and what only He can do for you. It demonstrates their distance and His nearness, their incompetence and His completeness, their one-sided knowledge and incomplete judgement and His perfect knowledge and inspection of you. Let this personal character of illness never be missed.

---

[13]See Appendix for the full text.

Every illness is a kind of chastisement and it comes home into the heart, saying *"You are the man!"* (2 Samuel 12:7). But the other view of it should never be forgotten.

Moreover, your illness is not for yourself alone, but for the whole Church *"...from whom the whole body, joined and held together by every joint with which it is equipped, when each part is working properly, makes the body grow so that it builds itself up in love"* (Ephesians 4:16). Those who are well could not go on without those who are ill, any more than those who are ill could go on without those who are well. In many things, the healthy need the sick.

They need to have this embodiment of a large part of the suffering of Jesus Christ kept constantly before them. They need to be reminded of death and Judgement. They need the ballast of suffering to keep them steady. They need to learn from it that *"Surely a man goes about as a shadow! Surely for nothing they are in turmoil; man heaps up wealth and does not know who will gather"* (Psalms 39:6).

They need that what is kind, sympathising and gentle in them to be developed and, through your own illness, refined. They need to see life real and in earnest with all its gloss stripped off, what it comes to, what they must come to. They need the voice of illness to say to them, *"Therefore you also must be ready, for the Son of Man is coming at an hour you do not expect"* (Matthew 24:44). To show them all this, is one purpose of illness.

If you look upon illness as a work, a mission to which God has called you, even though you seem only called to suffer, you will not look upon it as a lonely ordeal.

1.4 The Seeming Length of an Illness

A life-long illness? What a terrible thought. It seems as if it is going to be unending. But *"What is your life? You are you are a mist that appears for a little time and then vanishes"*

(James 4:14). Doctors may speak of its lasting indefinitely because its length cannot be defined by them.

With God are the issues of life and of death. He will daily and hourly, moment by moment, apportion to you your measure of suffering, as well as the measure of strength to carry you through it. You do not have to bear the whole length of your illness now, at this time, but only minute by minute. So do not increase your present suffering by adding to it the future burden. God knows how best to deal with you. Do not be afraid since all these things are in His hand and He lays them on you, not all at once, but little by little, to prepare you for greater tests.

We never have more a more severe trial than we can bear. We can always bear the present hour. For each day, so is our strength. If the trials of many years were gathered into one, we would be broken. Therefore, in compassion at our little strength, God sends first one and then another. Then he removes both and lays on a third, heavier perhaps, than either. But all pain is so wisely measured to our measure of strength that *"the bruised reed is never broken"*.

We must not look at our trials enough, in this continuous and successive view. Each test is sent to teach us something. Moreover, in total, they have a lesson which is beyond the power of any single one of them to teach on its own. If they came all at once and all together we should break down and learn nothing. The smoking flax would be put out and we should be crushed *"into the dust of death"* (Psalms 22:15). There is no other way to look at the path that lies in front of you. It seems a long and weary road without end. Or at least, the end is so far distant, so incalculable, that it seems endless.

You may have been told that your illness is not fatal, in itself, and yet it may last many years. But even imagining this is correct, it need not be this particular illness which is destined to remove you to the "rest that remains". Some other condition may come along any day and however slight it may seem, he who sends it can make it "his messenger" and it may bring the "true token" which is death.

Don't distress yourself, therefore, with trying to ascertain the probable length of your illness, the turns it might take, or how it may end. Leave everything to Him who said,*" I am the Way and the Truth and the Life*" (John 16:6). At the moment, you are saying with Thomas "*Lord, we do not know where you are going. How can we know the way?*" (John 14:5). The answer is the same, now as then "*I am the Way*". He is "the Way" in which you are walking. "The Truth" is your Teacher. "The Life" is Christ, in whom your life is hidden. To believe this, with your heart, would be perfect peace. You would have no second will of your own.

Allow God to lead you anywhere, through any illness, however long and wearisome it might be. Even though to you it seems to have no end, trust that it is the shortest, as well as the safest and the best way, the only way which can lead you where He has gone to prepare a place for you. By all these methods, He is preparing you for that place which He has already prepared for you. He knows exactly what is necessary.

On a dark night in a strange place, you must trust yourself to a guide. Put yourself into His hands. The way may seem very dark, dreary and solitary but He knows it. He has trodden every step and will surely lead you safely "*by a straight way till they reached a city to dwell in*" (Psalms 107:7).

1.5 Lessons which Various Illnesses are Meant to Teach

In the extreme of suffering from thirst which some have been called to pass through, when "*their tongue stuck to the roof of their mouth*" (Job 29:10) words failed "*my throat is parched*" (Psalms 69:3) and the spirit was faint from suffer-

Sickness: its Trials and Blessings

ing; in the peculiar distress of irritability and impatience which accompanies thirst, the restlessness, the fever, the feeling of intense misery, no one thinks it wrong to try and quench their thirst.

But when all help fails, then the spirit turns to God alone and gives thanks to Him who, when He was on the Cross, condescended to endure that suffering. Then those two words, *"I thirst"* (John 19:28) seemed inexpressibly gracious, loving and compassionate. They demonstrate His power to sympathise which has enabled many sufferers to lie still and bear His lesser woe. Those who, when they say "I am very thirsty" can quench the thirst. Those who when they are very hungry have food to eat and power to retain it, little know the exquisite tenderness of the loving-kindness of the Good Shepherd who suffered hunger and thirst for them.

Jesus Christ calls these sufferers to pass through these dry places, bears them in His arms, carries them in His bosom and leads them to see a fullness of meaning in the Gospels, which they could never have seen otherwise. For example, in the story of the miraculous loaves and fishes, He feeds many thousands with hardly any bread. It is not meaningless that three times in the year, the Church, in the Gospels appointed for Sundays, calls us to remember the miracle of the feeding of the five thousand.

The various forms of illness seem to teach us their own separate lesson *"Whoever is wise, let him attend to these things"* (Psalms 107:43)

- All those diseases which deprive people of some sense or power, speak each with their own voice and remind us that God gave us sight and hearing and the power of movement and action.

- Degenerative illnesses seem to say, perhaps with a louder voice than all the rest, "The Almighty God is the Lord of life and death and of all things which pertain to them".

- Those diseases which attack the digestive organs and which either prevent the digestion or the retaining of food, say that what we call 'common mercies' are the good gifts of God not once for all, but daily and hourly. We think it as a common mercy, if we regard it as a mercy at all, to be able to eat and, having eaten, to be nourished and suffer no inconvenience from it. We think it most odd if digestion is not like this, something that will quickly leave us. How many days, and months, and years, we have taken daily meals without looking at each one as a daily-renewed mercy from our ever watchful Lord, who *"knows our frame"* (Psalms 107:14)?

1.6 Sickness as a Vocation

Sickness for the moment is the state of life into which God has called you. It is your calling: your vocation. As such you will regard it as very good. You will also feel that no state can be as good as that to which He has called you. You will desire to have no choice about whether to live or to dies, to remain in your present state or to recover your physical health.

Whatever is clearly your work or your calling, do it! Be assured that we have no a *"hard man, reaping where you did not sow, and gathering where you scattered no seed"* (Matthew 25:24).

He will give you strength for each thing that He calls you to. But you must always remember that it is what He called you to and not any self-chosen path in which you cannot expect the power to perform your tasks. This is your work now and therefore do not scorn it. Do not disregard it or think of it lightly. This work requires great patience, great faith, great love and great submission. Ask yourself then, has He not honoured you by entrusting it to you?

Do you ask yourself how you can *"show forth His praise"* (Psalms 106:2) if you cannot move hand or foot, and I can scarcely think? The answer will give you work enough. For it will require a vigorous, earnest, daily, hourly, inner struggle, "a sharp rule over yourself", a true fight of faith which you cannot fight unless you *"take up the whole armour of God"* (Ephesians 6:13).

In some minds, there is a great impatience about the restrictions of sickness and an excessive desire for healing, which must be brought into subjection and yielded wholly to God. There are such a variety of characters and dispositions, that each person needs a different discipline.

Some learn more quickly in the school of sickness than others. Some make a great effort to learn and are never content with their present progress. They are always seeking to learn more, to practice more, to rise higher. This requires great self-discipline and constantly being on your guard. The birds of the air are constantly trying to eat the good seed sown on the ground and often the sun is very scorching. If the seed does not look for the dew which can moisten the ground, the ground becomes hard or the seed withers away.

Be careful about how you look upon yourself as cut off from life and from life's pleasures. You are not cut off, only taken aside, or "laid aside", possibly only for a short season or possibly for life. But you are still part of the Body of which Christ is the Head.

Some must suffer and some must serve, but each member is necessary to the others. *"The whole body is joined and held together by every joint with which it is equipped"* (Ephesians 4:16) *"The eye cannot say to the hand, I have no need of you nor again the head to the feet, I have no need of you"* (1 Corinthians 12:21).

Sickness: its Trials and Blessings

You may have been a very active person before your illness, or even an athlete: your life was filled with great energy and activity. Now you are grieving because you can no longer be busy, run or physically exercise. Do not grieve and do not envy those who can still do what you cannot. You may be given the work of the head or the eye, but the work is given by God. It may be the work of rest, of hardly moving hand or foot, scarcely speaking or showing any life, at all. Do not worry about it! If God has given it to you to do, it is His work and He will bless it.

Do not complain about it. Do not say "This is work, and this is not work". How do you know? What work do you think Daniel[14] was doing in the lions' den? Or Shadrach, Meshach, and Abednego in the fiery furnace? Their work was "glorious, laudable and honourable" for they were glorifying God in suffering.

If we truly knew what sorrow is, we should count it a high calling to be allowed to minister the least work of comfort to the afflicted. So, if we are called to suffer, let us understand it to be a call to a ministry of healing. God is setting us apart to a pastoral office, which is the care of the sick of His flock. There is a hidden ministry which works in perfect harmony with the orders of His Church. It is a ministry of secret comfort, diffusing itself by the power of sympathy and prayer.

Within His visible Church are many who sorrow, many who weep alone. It is a fellowship of secret mourners. To them, the contrite and humble in heart are perpetually ministering and shedding peace, though often unaware of it. Given in trust to them for the consolation of His elect, are the things they have learned in periods of suffering in their life and perceptions about God's love and presence. Often, they do not know where their words go. Perhaps they never see or ever will, in this life, those whom they have comforted? In fact, these chosen comforters may be unknown to one an-

---

[14]See Daniel Chapter 6

other, but they are bound together in bonds higher than blood bonds. They are joined and constituted in that higher unity which is the order of Christ's Kingdom so that when all the relationships in this lower life are dissolved, the bonds of their heavenly relationships will be revealed. Mourners and comforters will meet together in the holy City of God and *"He will wipe away every tear from their eyes, and death shall be no more, neither shall there be mourning, nor crying, nor pain any more, for the former things have passed away"* (Revelations 21.4).

You have been called to this ministry of healing. You have been set apart to perform it, through suffering. You learn how to fulfil it through the *"things which you suffer"* (Hebrews 5:8). You must go deep into the waters to feel how cold and deep they are and many times you thought you would be drowned, the *"deeps swallow me"* (Psalms 69:15). But you have been taught by suffering to know more of the Love and faithfulness of God than you could have learned in any other way.

Now you are called to go into the water with each person who asks for help and to show them that there is firm ground under their feet. You are called to show them where He is, He who though He appears to be sleeping only waits for them to cry to Him, *"Lord, save me or I perish"* (Matthew 8:25).

They may be trying to 'walk on the water' without having learned yet about human frailty. They are sinking and they cry to you for help[15]. Here is your work, delivered to your sick-bed. You asked for work and here is it. Be thankful for it and ask Him to bless it. Ask only to run your own race and to do your duty in the state of life in which it has pleased Him to call you. If you have been called to sickness, be joyful that you are considered *"worthy of this calling"* (2 Thessalonians 1:11) and *"submit yourself wholly to His holy will*

---

[15] See Matthew 14: 22-33.

and pleasure; and be sure that it shall turn to your profit, and help you forward in the right way that leads to everlasting life" (Service for the Visitation of the Sick).

1.7 The Probability of Recovery

Even if you consider your condition a life-long, chronic illness, there may be times when the possibility of recovery still seems reasonable. Sometimes, it may be with a sudden hope, with an impatient longing. At other times, with a hope that it will never happen, a rejection of the very idea of it. Then again, you may feel a morbid indifference or, yet again, a wild expectation.

Probably, when the illness started, you were willing either to die and go to be with the Lord[16], or desired for recovery and relief, with prayers, for recovery. Perhaps, you were almost frightened you would recover because you wanted to die so much. You were right to pray, in seriousness, that if it were the will of God, you would recover your bodily health. Health is a precious gift, full of blessings, responsibilities, sorrows and enjoyments. Besides, life is a wonderful and blessed gift from God and we ought to love life and heartily to give thanks for our "creation, preservation, and all the blessings of this life".

Perhaps your particular temptation has been not to value life enough, to be indifferent to it (and to health) and to see no brightness and blessing in it, only a depressing burden to be borne? You may have found it difficult to thank God for

---

[16]The Apostle Paul wrote: *"Yes, we are of good courage, and we would rather be away from the body and at home with the Lord. So whether we are at home or away, we make it our aim to please him"* (2 Corinthians 6:8,9); and: *"For to me to live is Christ, and to die is gain. If I am to live in the flesh, that means fruitful labour for me. Yet which I shall choose I cannot tell. I am hard pressed between **the two**. My desire is to depart and be with Christ, for that is far better. But to remain in the flesh is more necessary on your account. Convinced of this, I know that I will remain and continue with you all, for your progress and joy in the faith."* (Philippians 1: 21-25)

your "creation and preservation". At times, sinfully, you have wished your days on earth were over. You have believed that you are ready to die, or at least you felt that God could make you ready at any moment. Instead of "seeing the balance of good and evil", your years have been those in which you said," *I have no pleasure in them*" (Ecclesiastes 12:1).

You have carried <u>your weary load of discontent</u> with life, and have envied the dead who have escaped from it. You thought that you wished to "*...to depart and be with Christ, for that is far better*" (Philippians 1:23). But perhaps you are really more anxious to escape duties, from inner conflicts, from pain and depression? How often you have said, "*Oh, that I had wings like a dove! I would fly away and be at rest*" (Psalms 55:6)? You could not enjoy life: you refused to. You had much to make it pleasant but you would not look at the bright things and thought there was nothing but darkness around you.

You thought, for example, that you were not treated lovingly enough by others, or that everyone you have loved best had been taken from you or that your closest emotional bonds had been cut and you were being called to go on living. You cannot say from your heart "God is Love," or rather "Love" to you. You felt that He dealt harshly with you. If you were ill, you impatiently watched your symptoms hoping that each one was fatal. You were angry when friends said that you were getting or looking better and even more angry if a doctor said so. You thought they did not know and understand because you preferred to die, but you were being compelled to go on living. Your spirit fretted at what seemed an unreasonable delay, such a long time to wait to escape.

You may have often prayed for a ministry and yet, when you have been given it, it has not seemed enough for your capacities. Or it is not the kind suited to you. So your soul has never been at rest, because it has constantly been feeling after something that it has never found.

Part II - ASPECTS OF ILLNESS

2.1 Pain

People often ask whether pain or weakness is the hardest to bear? Some of the chronically ill speak of one as much easier to bear than the other. However, in a long illness they are possibly almost inseparable. They are so intermixed together that it is scarcely possible to say which kind of suffering is to be classed under each heading.

There are pains which are distinct from weakness and weakness is not always accompanied by pain. Those words, "It is just weakness" and "It is only weakness" are as despairing as any words that can be uttered in a long and weary condition. No matter whether there is a clear reason for weakness or not, the trial is the same.

Some people are endowed with much more natural courage and fortitude than others. For them, it is not so difficult to bear acute pain for a short time. But when it is drawn out, when it requires patience, patience and fortitude are not always combined.

There is a peculiar character in severe chronic pain when it first happens. It seems to bring all the sins of our lives before us and to "speak to us with a piercing emphasis". We cannot understand it. The nature of pain is quite incomprehensible and its effects are hidden from us. We do not see its prognosis, so how can we know its object? If we think about the incomprehensible nature of pain, mental and bodily, we must consider its hidden nature, its vividness, its penetration and its omnipresence in our whole being. If we think about its inscrutable origin, we must think about the indissoluble link which binds it to original sin. Then, we must consider its mysterious relation to the Cross, the Passion and perfection of our Lord. Then we shall see reason to believe that a power so near and so awful has much energy, and fulfils many designs in God's kingdom, which are secret.

Some pains are much more difficult to bear than others. For example:

- those which affect the head and prevent all mental activity;
- some internal pains that have a knife-like sharpness;
- some diseases that are contagious or physically unsightly and it requires an effort of love or duty to nurse them and they involve so much inexpressible and inconceivable suffering that life becomes mere endurance.

These, and many other conditions, such as constant nausea and inability to retain food teach us that these are "bodies of humiliation". They help us to take hold of and understand something of the wonderful meaning and blessing of Jesus' promise, *"But our citizenship is in heaven, and from it we await a Saviour, the Lord Jesus Christ, who will transform our lowly body to be like his glorious body, by the power that enables him even to subject all things to himself"* (Philippians 3:20-21).

There is a large class of hidden emotional and physical pains which gain no sympathy whatsoever, and yet which cause great suffering to those who have them.

A chronic condition may be something quite straightforward but it will not respond to treatment. It may be some mysterious or little understood condition. It may be something hidden which doctors can neither explain nor remove, but which may as effectually 'scourge' the sufferer as any knotted cord could scourge it. We think of it as a pain without glory, because bearing it in a cheerful spirit brings no honour or credit. The pain goes on and on and there is no improvement in it. Years pass and it is still there, as fresh to you in its suffering as when it first began, but the novelty has gone. The vigorous effort of patience is over. It wears you out, day by day. Your friends have mostly forgotten it. Now and then, someone asks whether you still suffer from it and you feel that it is very kind of them to remember. But, for the most part, the tale of your suffering is forgotten, and you must bear it alone, as far as those near you are concerned.

You may have seen many doctors and specialists[17]. Some see nothing in it worth interest. Others for lack of a better name call it a "nervous" complaint. Some tell you that there is no treatment and it will remain with you as long as you live. Well, so be it! No length of years or continuance of pain will ever cause Him who sends the condition or pain to forget your suffering or that you cannot bear it for a moment, without His help.

God who appoints the length and measure of the suffering, does not send it and forget what He has done and how He has caused you to suffer. He will be near you because it is His "visitation". The only fear is that you forget that He is near, do not know or realise His presence, nor ask His help, but think instead that you can bear it all alone. If you do so, then you will cease to be able to bear it and will become *"like an untrained calf"* (Jeremiah 31:18).

Ask Him to give you that living faith which sees His hand bringing the condition and fitting it in all its minutest parts to your character and needs. He holds it so that it does not press too heavily even on the tenderest parts, to enable you to see how it is working for you. This is a far more exceeding and eternal weight of glory. This faith would enable you to see *"an eternal weight of glory beyond all comparison, as we look not to the things that are seen but to the things that*

---

[17]This is reminiscent of the women who comes to Jesus in Mark, *"who had suffered much under many physicians, and had spent all that she had, and was no better but rather grew worse"* (Mark 5:26).

are unseen. For the things that are seen are transient, but the things that are unseen are eternal"* (2 Corinthians 4:17-18).

Do not try to measure or compare pain. For example, do not compare your pain with that of others, asking whether it is greater or less than someone else's or than a pain that you have suffered in the past. Simply bear it, as it is, not as you think it could be modified. Do not be too eager and restless to get it relieved or removed. Until it is the will of God that it is removed, bear it silently, patiently, *"rendering service with a good will as to the Lord and not to man"* (Ephesians 6:7).

Look to Jesus Christ for the blessing from it, and you will receive it. At times, it may seem almost impossible to bear this pain any longer. In fact, it would be impossible to bear, if the bearing of it was yours alone, but *"He gives us more grace"* (James 4:6). *"He took our illnesses and bore our sicknesses"* (Matthew 8:17).

God knows the measure and the number of your pains. *"In all their affliction he was afflicted, and the angel of his presence saved them; in his love and in his pity he redeemed them; he lifted them up and carried them all the days of old"* (Isaiah 63:9). He will carry you now, and to the end of your illness, however distant that hour and day may be.

2.2 Weakness

Weakness forms a great part of all illnesses of whatever kind. It is a state full of distress and temptations. To each one of us it seems to be *"a wilderness, a land of deserts and pits, a land of drought and deep darkness, in a land that none passes through, where no man dwells"* (Jeremiah 2:6). However, *"a great multitude that no one could number, from every nation, from all tribes and peoples and languages"* (Revelations 7:9) are walking there, continually, each one of them thinking that he or she is walking alone.

Sickness: its Trials and Blessings

The Variation of Weakness in Different People

Weakness and debility differ so much in their intensity, and in their condition, that no one can measure them in another person.

Even the sick often misunderstand and misjudge weakness in each other and think that because one person who is ill can do certain things, everyone else can. This is a universal mistake relating to weakness.

Weakness affects people in very different ways, differing according to the disease and according to the patient's physical make-up and constitution. For example,

- one person may not be able to leave his bed;
- another, may not be at all less really ill, yet may be able to get up and walk around the house, can bear to go out and perhaps even might go for a short walk;
- another may be unable to bear to see even a close friend or talk at all and yet may be able to get up and get dressed;
- another sufferer, may be unable to talk;
- another might be able to write;
- another is unable to read or use their mind in any way, without the most painful results.

The first person may be able to bear a great deal of noise, another, none at all. Extreme nervous agitation of the mind may be produced by traffic or noises in the house or internal noise like a door slammed, a loud tone of voice, or even the voice of a child. Another may like to have a light room because it is cheerful and yet another may not be able to bear light at all. The latter may be unable to bear a voice reading aloud, while the former may enjoy it and find it very soothing. To some, the effort of concentration may be impossible; to others, it may be easier to read to oneself or to talk to someone. Yet in reality the latter group may not be more ill than the former.

Weakness shows itself in very different ways. Therefore *"Judge not, that you be not judged"* (Matthew 7:1) but leave it all to Him who is *"a righteous judge, strong and patient"* (Psalms 7:11).

The Problem of Sensitivity to Light

It is quite certain that of the many forms of trial and temptations presented by weakness, each one has to be fought and resisted, but quietly. Otherwise annoyance will increase and then the trial would be all but impossible to overcome.

If noises distress you, remember that by giving into your nervous irritation and in removing every cause of noise as far as it is possible, you put yourself more into the position of being worn down by it. If, instead of having everyone come into your room or walk about the house on tip-toe, you try to get used to the sound of their natural step, it will prevent much ongoing distress.

If you try to bear irritations, gradually you will find that you mind them, less and less. If, when children or teenagers are around, you tell them to go away or be quiet, you deprive them of much pleasure in coming to see you. You will make their visits inhibited and unpleasant and deprive yourself of the enjoyment of them and their love and enjoyment of their individual characters. You will give them the impression, perhaps for life, that disability and illness creates a depressing atmosphere, to be avoided, only to be visited out of necessity. You little know the negative effect that this impression may have on them, or the opposite impression, for their good. For their sake, they should be reminded that with someone who is ill they must be quieter than elsewhere and that they should not be boisterous. They should be taught from an early age to respect and consider the poor, for *"In the day of trouble the Lord delivers him"*[18].

For your own sake, never become too selfish about noise, light, or anything else if you can prevent yourself. The ability to bear things increases with habit and with determination. But, if the temptation is yielded to, the power, or the supposed capability, diminishes, until finally you will become really incapable of bearing almost anything.

The Problem of Sensitivity to External Noises

You can never get rid of all external noises, for example traffic, building works and so on. They are the most difficult of any noises to get used to. In certain states, they can be very distressing and seem to become more painful and less bearable, as time goes by.

The only solution is to tell yourself, "I am placed here by God. He put me here, in this very place, to work for him. If I try to escape from the noise, I shall disobey Him. It is meant to test my faith and complete obedience. He, I know, will help me to bear it, minute by minute. It is all His will."

Of course, there are states of physical suffering, in which noise and light must, as far as possible, be shut out, for a time but they are the exceptions. Here we are speaking of ordinary, everyday cases of background noise.

The Habits of Illness

In every way, the fewer invalid habits you develop in illness and disability, the better it will be for you in the long run, for your health and happiness, and that of all those around

---

[18] Psalms 41:1. This verse bears an important message for carers of the disabled, sick and weak. A compassionate God will see all compassionate actions towards the weak and broken in body, heart and mind (whether they are Christians or non-Christians) and will protect, preserve and bless them "in the land". We must assume that caring for the weak, in some mysterious way, protects carers from evil.

you. These habits grow quickly in the sick and they have to be resisted in the earliest stages.

A sick person should try to consider as few things necessary as possible and to deny himself or herself in little things, so that selfishness does not start to grow. In illness, you have a real battle on your hands not to become moody, morbid, self-centred, inconsiderate and totally insensitive to everyone around you.

Weakness of Mind

You often feel as if you were imprisoned by physical suffering. You may have a heavy burden of constant malaise, depression and pain, in a state in which your mind has been much weakened. It is so difficult to focus your thoughts on anything. You try to but the mental effort seems to increase your mental and physical weakness. Your mind seems unable to fix on anything. You may try to think. You think of a topic, but you say, "What was I thinking about? My mind is confused, muddled and weak". Don't try too hard. Let your thoughts go. *"As water spilled on the ground"* (Genesis 38:9 AV) so are they.

Do not distress yourself about not being able to think clearly. It is all part of being ill. You must be passive now and let Him work on your behalf. Ask God to *"put into your mind good desires"* (Collect for Easter Day). It is only by "His holy inspiration that we think those things that are good" (Collect for Fifth Sunday after Easter). Lie back and rest in him, and if we may say it, reverently of course, let Him "do the thinking" for you.

Mental and Spiritual Warfare

You may be beset by constantly going over bad experiences in your mind and by forgetting all your happiest memories. You may have been exposed to some trauma which, for the entire world, you wish you had spared. Yet now, in your mental weakness, such things are set lose to haunt and torment you and threaten to put you in the grip of a severe temptation to despair. This is, in fact, a very difficult trial of faith but a very common one.

Satan takes advantage of our mental weakness. There can be no doubt in that. But there is One who is stronger than the Enemy, who will not let you be tempted beyond what you can bear.

> *"No temptation has overtaken you that is not common to man. God is faithful, and he will not let you be tempted beyond your ability, but with the temptation he will also provide the way of escape, that you may be able to endure it."* (1 Corinthians 10:13)

Our Lord, who was severely tempted by the Adversary, knows your deepest feelings. He was not only tempted, but also overcame the devil. And He overcame him, for your sake.

Resisting the Devil in Illness

The devil and sin *"will have no dominion over you, since you are not under law but under grace"* (Romans 6:14). Even so, do not wage war on temptation alone. Don't struggle with the Enemy in your own strength, or he will tempt you further. Just say, *"Get behind me, Satan! For you are not setting your mind on the things of God"* (Mark 8:33). Do not listen. Petition God, as if no voices of temptation were in your ears. If they still drown out *"the voice of your petition, cry out to God even more."* (Luke 22:44) Jesus who wrestled with Satan was in an agony of sweat. Your agony will never be as great as His, but you need simply to cry out: "By your Cross and saving blood, good Lord, deliver me."

Remember that Jesus is near, empathizing with you and strengthening you. Do not dispute with yourself or with

Satan. Do not analyse your thoughts. Do not say, "Where did this idea come from?".

There is no safe path through temptation, by just thinking about it. Simply shut your ears and carry on crying out to God. This trial may return, often. Do not imagine that when the battle seems won, it will not begin again. But its power over you will steadily weaken if you treat it like this, until finally the Enemy will leave you, but only for a period. Finding that particular weakness in your armour is protected by the blood of Christ, he will look for some other vulnerable place to attack you.

Do not torment yourself by thinking how much more evil your thoughts are than they used to be. There is no proof that this is the case. Satan made evil suggestions to our Lord and *"A disciple is not above his teacher, but everyone when he is fully trained will be like his teacher."* (Luke 6:40) Do not dwell on it. In your weak state, it will only increase the evil in your trial.

If you resist a temptation, instantaneously, it does not become sin but only a bitter trial and struggle. If you think about it too deeply and turn it over too much in your mind, more than your weakness wants you to do, you will turn it into a sin. You must meet the trial with the only safe words to meet all trials: "This trial is the will of God."

Evil Desires in Illness

Similarly, resist all evil thoughts which come into your mind. Evil will come in the form of:

- irritability;
- impatience;
- discontent;
- rebellious thoughts against God;
- inordinate craving for sympathy;

- fear;
- despair at endless suffering;
- fear of <u>social isolation</u>;

Without doubt, these are very difficult trials to bear, especially as in illness they often attract not only little or no compassion, and even aggravation from others. This attitude stems not only from unkindness and hardness of heart but also from ignorance and thoughtlessness. It is so difficult in weakness to hold up the shield of faith against these *"flaming darts of the evil one"* (Ephesians 6:16), the shield which alone can keep them from entering the soul.

Getting confused in what you say

Another trial in weakness is the difficulty of finding the right words, the words you intended. You know perfectly what word you want to say and then you say another which means something completely different.

You ask to have something given to you which is different from what you want. Or you say what you do not intend and so do not get the thing which you want.

This is very trying, but it stems from physical weakness. Do not be distressed or depressed by muddling your words. It will pass away when you get better or stronger. In the meantime, see it as a way of humbling you, intellectually. Instead of being upset and annoyed at it, just say, "This is God's will".

The Unknown and Foreign Nature of Illness

You cannot know a foreign country unless you have either been there or read descriptions of it, and tried to imagine the place.

No one who has not had sickness themselves or has not carefully watched those who are sick, can have any idea of the real state of illness[19]. Friends do not see you after one of their visits, which for the time you may have really needed and enjoyed, but which leave you quite exhausted. For a few hours, you can do nothing, neither read nor think. Then perhaps you start to read something or do something, but after a little while, exhaustion overtakes you.

This is how you spend each day. Every exertion is followed by periods of rest. Your time is not only all broken up but your strength can never be relied on because your strength varies from day to day. Sometimes the whole day is spent in a state barely removed from unconsciousness, if that means being half able to understand what is happening, because you are deeply conscious of a weary tiredness and an inner exhaustion which is quite unutterable.

Or, your time may be spent in merely bearing pain, taking treatment, and then in resting afterwards. You may feel feverish or restless: your need and treatment is to rest completely, to lie perfectly still, without moving or doing anything. Or some particular pain or mental suffering may be increased by every single activity and you are doomed to total boredom for most of the day. On top of this, your life is so dependent on others.

People who are well, if they want or need to be alone, can go out for a walk or go into another room - but you cannot. Where you are, you have to remain. You must put up with whoever comes in and stays for as long as they like. However unwilling you are to be interrupted in what you are concentrating on doing, you must receive it as 'discipline' and not discourage your visitor, in case next time he or she will feel that he was in your way and not come at all. This 'being at the mercy of others' and your inability to shut

---

[19] This is also why direct experience of suffering often makes us into 'broken healers', more competent in understanding and comforting others: "[God] *who comforts us in all our affliction, so that we may be able to comfort those who are in any affliction, with the comfort with which we ourselves are comforted by God*" (2 Corinthians 1:4).

anyone out or even to lock the door, is a constant trial to the sick.

You may have much too much spare time, but the energy to use it constructively is rarely given to you. Even when it seems to be, or when by sheer willpower, you try to push yourself beyond your weakness, then you alone know the suffering it causes. You know the painful effort at the time and the extreme distress which follows. There is the extreme discouragement of relapsing and the sense of annihilation of mind. The life of your body seems to consist of misery, helplessness and suffering. Every nerve fibre seems on edge and every nerve-ending is calling out to you in a voice of anguish.

You hear a bell ring, a footstep on the stairs or a knock at the door and you desperately hope that no one is coming near you to make demands in your extreme weakness. You feel that you could be rude to anyone who talks to you. You have just time to cry out: Lord, help me! *"Be gracious to me, O LORD, for I am languishing; heal me, O Lord, for my bones are troubled"* (Psalms 6:2) when someone enters your room. Well, don't fear what feels like intrusion. Carry on saying those words in your own heart. God will help you and you will *"never be put to shame"* (1 Peter 2:6).

Your visitor leaves you. You realise that you have, thanks to God, been enabled to avoid expressing your suffering, though you think that your tone or manner showed it. You feel that even if you managed to avoid saying anything which might be sinful, sin was in your heart.

Then you feel crushed and depressed because you know that secretly, irritability and impatience were present. The nervous irritability, unutterable in its extent, causes you a continual and bitter conflict inside in order to hold it down, even to avoid it showing outwardly. *"Be still before the LORD and wait patiently for him; fret not yourself over the one who prospers in his way, over the man who carries out evil devices"*

(Psalms 37:7) is the only thing for you to do in such testing circumstances.

One week, you may greatly dread hearing the sound of footsteps or someone calling you. Then, next week, your trial is that you have been lying alone for too long. You feel you have reactive depression. You feel *"I have been forgotten like one who is dead; I have become like a broken vessel"* (Psalms 31:12).

You may have been thinking of your loneliness and of your chronic condition as you suppose it to be. You may have been aware of your inability to do the many things that you longed to do. You may dread the future which seems dark, empty and full of boredom. You may miss friends who have passed into Eternity, who have understood you and who would have sympathized with you.

Now you are left alone and without comfort. Then you imagine that you are a burden and a trouble to everyone, a person without meaning, except for the trouble you give them. You go on, perhaps, to think that they do not love you. You feel isolated, depressed and lonely, and ask, *"O Lord, how long?"* (Psalms 6:3).

Then, someone visits or calls you. Maybe it is one of the family who just looked in to say some kind word or to bring you a book to interest you. Or you receive an interesting communication, book or letter, or a flower, or a message from some friend. Maybe, it is only an often unvalued message of love : "So-and-so sends her love to you", but it is enough. The whole tenor of your thoughts changes and you see how unfairly you have accused your family and friends of indifference and see that the isolation and lack of love was in you, not in them. In this way, you feel cheered and replenished as you carry on, refreshed. Sometimes even someone coming into the room on some errand will be sufficient to divert your thoughts into a fresh channel.

Sickness: its Trials and Blessings

If your friends could really read your thoughts and see the change in them, what an effort they would make to give you messages, however trifling, *"to let you know you are remembered and still kept in the unity of the Church"* (Service for the Visitation of the Sick).

How much they want to bring you little "gifts of time and pleasure". They would feel, too, that when they visit you, they should be interesting in their conversation generally, because you need to have the current of your thoughts changed and stimulated and because you have so painful a sense of weakness, that, apart from the effort to rouse yourself, you feel you can offer them nothing.

Never forget that Jesus knows all about your weakness. *"For he knows our frame; he remembers that we are dust"* (Psalms 103:14).

Be confident that when you pray, *"Be gracious to me, O Lord, for I am languishing; heal me, O Lord, for my bones are troubled"* (Psalms 6:2), you will always be heard. You can be sure that although *"As for me, I am poor and needy, but the Lord takes thought for me. You are my help and my deliverer ; do not delay, O my God!"* (Psalms 40:17).

2.3 Loss of the Powers of the Mind

The Church has classed age, weakness, and sickness together (Service for the Visitation of the Sick) since these trials are in many respects, the same.

In many ways, the beautiful description of age in Ecclesiastes Chapter 12 applies to your state[20]. The years have already come (they no longer "coming") when you say, "I have no

---

[20] This passage talks about old age, about the keepers of the house trembling, doors to a street being closed, the sound of work fading and songs growing faint. Old people become afraid of heights and of dangers in the street. It is a time when desire is no longer aroused. Priscilla Maurice compares this state with illness.

pleasure in them". "The sun and the light and the moon and the stars" have grown dark for you. They have lost their brightness. The clouds return after the rain. They gather again when they seem to have dispersed and, as yet, you *"see not the bright light, the sun, that there is in the sky after the wind has swept the skies clean"* (Job 37:21). The keepers of the house tremble and the strong men stoop". Those "looking through the windows grow dim". Likewise, your mind and judgement have strangely aged: they are strangely weakened.

In health, you almost used to pride yourself on the rapidity with which you came to decisions. Now, it is only slowly and unwillingly that you can take decisions. One moment the decision is made and the next, a host of fears overturn it, or at least shake your confidence. You, who used to despise asking for help, in even the slightest things or even in great things, now turn to others to ask for help, or rather to decide, instead of yourself. They don't see or seem to see, the doubts in your mind and all the implications. You are dissatisfied with their decision : it will not do. So you must decide for yourself, deeply aware that your own vision is disturbed and darkened, and that you have lost confidence in balancing things.

Then, after you make a decision, misgivings follow. Perhaps I was wrong? Would it have been better to have decided this or that? Is it too late to change your mind? Then, maybe, you find it is.

Do not let it worry you : our first thoughts are often the truest and wisest and when we indulge in second thoughts we often make mistakes and return to the initial ones. The truth is that your judgement is simply not to be trusted now. It is affected by the general weakness of your body. Be confident, however, that if you commit it and yourself to the *"Lord of hosts, who judges righteously"* (Jeremiah 11:20). *"He leads the humble in what is right, and teaches the humble his way"* (Psalms 25:9).

If you trust him to decide, you will not go wrong. The less you complain about it, the better. Those who are ill are the most deeply conscious of their own failure of mental power, of the unreliability of their judgement and perception and indeed, they are the very people who make the best counsellors and make the wisest decisions. This is because they go outside themselves and their own powers and rely for everything on *"the Wonderful Counsellor"* (Isaiah 9:6), speaking his words (using Scripture) rather than their own.

It seems that a heavenly instinct is given to the sick : *"The friendship of the Lord is for those who fear him, and he makes known to them his covenant"* (Psalms 25:14).

Grief over Mental Losses in Illness

Do not mourn the loss of anything now lost which was merely your own capacity, or which you used to think was yours. *"God had provided something better for us, that apart from us they should not be made perfect"* (Hebrews 11:40). This something is fullness of grace. So thank God in advance for his gifts and he will give them to you richly.

Loss of Memory

What we have said about judgement can also be said about memory, in illness. Do not think your trial peculiar to yourself alone if you find that you have lost your memory.

Memory loss is one of the most likely accompaniments of weakness. Memory depends mainly on the state of health. It will probably gradually return and regain its power, if you recover your physical strength. Memory varies too, even in weakness, from day to day, often being merely related to the state of the stomach or nerves. It fails in different ways and degrees in different individuals:

- some will lose the power remember the little things of everyday life; their minds will be tormented if anyone asks them to remember anything, or expects them to remind someone else about it.
- others will lose all memory of names or dates.
- others will have a exactness of memory about dates and names and yet will be frustrated if others do not remember things as well as they do, and as minutely, or in the same way as they do.
- others, cannot recall anything that they read, however deeply it interests them.
- to some, remembering a fact in history, or life, however well known in the past, is an impossibility.
- others will lose all verbal memory and can scarcely even repeat words after someone else has said them.
- some may have stores of poetry in their minds, which now they cannot access or lay hold of.

In some cases, there will be many of these types of memory loss occurring together at the same time. Some people are especially tested by an inability to repeat, or remember words of Scripture correctly, or to recall hymns or creeds with which they were very familiar. Sometimes they cannot finish The Lord's Prayer, or even the 23rd Psalm. This loss is very depressing at first and the more so because "we are not unaware of Satan's schemes (96)", that Satan may try to persuade the sufferer that this proves that he or she does not value the words of Scripture any more.

The remedies for this trial of memory are:
- Do not burden your memory at all, but write everything down. Do this with all little tasks and with messages. Never try to remember them, but keep your mind free and unfettered for better thoughts.

- Never strain the memory, or over-tax it. Be content now to remember one text, instead of many sentences.
- Try and learn some little verse from the Scriptures, or poetry, each day, just enough to keep the memory a little exercised.
- Do not think about loss of memory. Try to act and speak as you used to do, without prefacing your words or thoughts with how you have "lost your memory".
- When it is worst, do not worry yourself by grieving over it as this will increase the evil effects of the memory loss.
- Remember always who has sent you this trial. God knows that it belongs to your weakness and how trying it is. He judges you with justice and does not think that you love the Bible less, because you cannot recall it correctly and have forgotten much of it.

All this is very humbling because you cannot appear as you might like to, in front of your friends. You cannot enter into conversation with the same pleasure to yourself, or to others. You feel that you are a shadow or wreck of your former self.

All this God sees, knows and feels. But He sees that this trial is necessary or He would not have sent it. He will fulfil His promise that *"the Counsellor, the Holy Spirit will teach you all things and remind you of everything I have said to you"*[21]. Be sure that nothing will be lost. Whatever you need *"...for teaching, for reproof, for correction and for training in righteousness, that the man of God may be competent, equipped for*

---

[21] John 14:26. Priscilla Maurice slightly misapplies this text. The original was addressed by Jesus to His disciples, assuring them that they would recall what He has said to them. There is no reference in the Biblical text that this applies to sufferers in illness.

every good work" (2 Timothy 3:16-17) can be brought to your mind and taught to you.

Often, those who feel most that their memory is failing, seem to learn most freshly and most vividly truths which they perhaps knew before, but have forgotten. Now these truths strike them afresh with new depth and with a meaning never perceived before.

In suffering, God, Himself, is teaching them. Sometimes indeed, a truth will come back with such a startling clarity that we think we can never forget it. Yet just an hour later we cannot even remember what the subject of it was! We make efforts to pursue and recapture the thought but in vain. It has not really gone. It has only sunk into our hearts, become a part of ourselves, and laid up safely by Him who brought it to us. He knows where it is and when to direct us to it, when we need it again. Let us *"commit the keeping of our memories, like our souls to Him "a faithful Creator"* (1 Peter 4:19). When the sad thought of loss of one's memory returns, say *"It is the will of God"*. This alone can silence your complaint.

Inability to Talk

You may have difficulty in holding a conversation. You feel either that you have knowledge that would not interest others or else that from illness and loneliness, you have lost the power to think, talk and understand. You imagine that you cannot interest others or will look unintelligent through the feebleness of your mind, which you know is a shadow of what it once was.

When you hear new issues discussed, you feel, "This is quite beyond me. How I used to join in with lively interest! I used to grasp and understand ideas, but now it all seems in a foreign language which I cannot understand. I can't follow the words and concepts at all. I shall make strange stupid mistakes if I join in and if anyone asks me to summarise what

Sickness: its Trials and Blessings

has been said, I would hardly know. Yet I used to be so familiar with this subject".

This is a peculiarly distressing feeling. The more you focus on it, the stronger the sense of inadequacy becomes. Finally, you start thinking you cannot even understand adult sentence and thoughts and that children's literature is all that remains for you.

Why not tell your friends that you cannot understand them, but not in a complaining, fretful tone. Let them carry on normally and you will glean something, if you are patient. Do not inwardly torture yourself because you cannot cope with the supposed humiliation.

The best thing to do when these thoughts start up again is to say to yourself, "Well, what can I do about it? I will just have to listen, join in the conversation whenever I can. Some ideas I can understand. The rest I cannot follow at all because my mind is so weak". Who has taken your power of understanding away? In complaining and self-torment, who are you rebelling against? It is God who has permitted it.

The same applies to reading aloud. If you are asked by a friend if you would like to hear a reading, you can answer according to your preferences and ability. But if you are well enough to join in with the family and they are reading some book, do not ask them to change it, or not to read, merely became you have this feeling of an inability to understand or because a continuous voice annoys you and prevents you staying focused (which to some of the sick is always the case with reading aloud).

Enter with cheerfulness and willingness into their pleasure and tell your pain only to Him who sees your heart. Then you will surely have gained by it yourself, in patience, humility and charity. Take every opportunity of trying to overcome the great difficulty which you feel in taking an interest in other people's concerns and in the things which interest them. It is a trial common to sickness but should be earnestly resisted, and may be wonderfully overcome.

2.4 The Nearness of Life

When, at first, the sense of being so close to life and yet it is out of reach comes upon you, it is a very hard test. The sick person vainly hopes to become used to it, but do not be deceived: this feeling will never diminish its power over you.

One day you imagine that you have got used to it. Then some little thing happens which reveal the whole sad truth and you may find yourself just where you were. You say, "There is only one step between me and life". But that step! How can it be taken?

A few feet may separate you from your family. You hear their voices and laughter. At times you catch their words. Then family prayers begin. Once you did not value them but now, how gladly you would hear them. But those few feet shut out all but the occasional sound of a word.

Someone else visits the family, just as you begin to imagine that you are reconciled to your circumstances. This person is more to you than to them and the tone of their voice ascends, but that is all. Perhaps you will not even meet them. At any rate, you will forfeit their company.

Or, perhaps, for a time you have moved to the house of some friend and you long very much to share in all their activities and pleasures. You faintly, dimly hear what is going on, but you are shut off from the sight and enjoyment of their life. You share it only during their occasional, perhaps rare, visits.

You have a new lesson to learn as there is nothing that so effectively tempts and tests a sick person. This is this trial: to seem to be separated from our companions tends to lead us into most untrue and hard thoughts about them. When you hear a bell ring to call the family together for a meal, you long to be there at the table and you think how much you are deprived of their company. You think about how much you would love to be with them, how much news and conversation you are missing, how many things you should like to hear and to ask and to say!

Bear it always in mind that you are now, by the will of God, brought into a different state from them, different from your former state; that you are called to new duties and responsibilities, comforts, blessings, trials and temptations. And who called you? It is God.

2.5 Longings

Many desires for that which you do not have, or cannot have, often come into your mind and sometimes they seem very painful. You sense that these desires are wrong and resist them. But then, at another time, you feel as if they ought to be fulfilled for you, as if your friends should try to give them to you. You think that they *must* know you want them, that they *must* realize how great a pleasure this or that would be to you.

Ask yourself, "Is this reasonable?" To give an example: if you are unable to move, the longing for the relief which would given to you by crossing the room they surely cannot be expected to understand? They can move whenever, and as freely they want to, scarcely seeming to will it.

Fully to understand this, one must have spent many weary months in the same position. It is not love of change that causes the desire to move. It is the peculiar relief produced by it. The very movement through the air seems to change the thoughts and throw off some sad feelings which are very hard to shake off when circumstances are unchanged because they seem to settle down and fasten upon the weak body and to press upon the weakened mind. *"For the corruptible body is a load upon the soul and the earthly habita-*

tion presses down the mind that muses upon many things" (Wisdom 9:15).

You see life as one shut in by four walls, each wall having its own peculiar pictures on it. Do not expect those whose hands have never painted them, to see them? Neither the pictures, nor their black frames will be visible to their eyes. Do not expect it this perception from other people : accept that it is unreasonable.

The bright lights of nature will perhaps never brighten those framed pictures for you. But there is a brighter Light that can illuminate them everything and change them all into "pleasant" pictures.

Do not condemn your friends as selfish if they cannot understand your profound and irrepressible longing to see all the things in which you have so intensely delighted. You may be burning with a wasting desire just to see a field, to wander deep in a wood, or even under a few trees, in a wheat-field, across a meadow with cattle grazing, or to see a river or flowers growing.

You may repress the longing to all outward observers. You may never express it and there may even be a sense of mournful submission about it, a sense that not seeing it is "all right". And yet, at times, the pain of longing may be intense. It may suddenly seize you and it seems as if you had no strength to grapple with it. You feel you must see these things, whatever happens. You think you can concentrate on nothing, until your desire is granted.

You mention it to a friend. It is treated at first, perhaps, as mere nonsense and you are counted very foolish for wishing for impossibilities and not submissive enough to God's will for desiring anything you cannot have. You say in your heart (and thank God if you do not say any reproachful words aloud), "How selfish it is of those who have all these enjoyments not in the least to enter into my desires, and only to throw them back on me!"

Sickness: its Trials and Blessings

You turn inward into yourself and no longer speak about your longings. But there they are. They burn and well-nigh consume you. No one who has not experienced this, can explain the trial of these desires or the sudden way in which they will come upon a sick person. One moment one may think that that one is quite used to one's lot; the next, a desire may shoot across the heart which may show how far this is from being attained.

Yet do not be discouraged. These are only temptations and if rightly treated, they may never pass into sin, but rather, gradually, strengthen your submission. Only do not expect those who have never experienced such a test to understand it. People generally imagine that if a person is confined for years to bed, all these trials must be overcome and belong to an early stage of illness. But this is not true. After ten years or more of such confinement, after even the sufferer himself has looked upon such internal conflict as ended, the flame may suddenly and cause great distress.

These longings come in various ways and each season brings its own peculiar temptations. Perhaps the greatest time of trial is the spring. As each spring returns, the same fight seems to need to be fought all over again. The trees begin to bud and the almond-tree blossoms and to some sick people it brings more hope and pleasure than any other blossom of the year. "The trees are bursting, and here am I still in my bed". No change in me except that of increased suffering, weakness and weariness.

The air is getting fresher and more free: *"The flowers appear on the earth, the time of singing has come, and the voice of the turtle-dove is heard in our land"* (Song of songs 2:12). Their voices are very joyous, but I can scarcely think obvious. They seem to tell how free and blithe they are and can fly whither they will, but I am: "a prisoner and a captive."

Other people can go out into the fresh air and they come in and enjoy saying how tired they are. "Oh! How much I should enjoy everything if I could go out". The trees put forth their leaves, and *"you know that summer is near"* (Matthew 24:32). Each day the poor, sick person grows at first more and more excited, and then finally, more and more depressed. "It is this season in which I must go out", they think. Autumn will come soon and I cannot go out then. It will be too chilly and damp and the trees will be losing their summer brightness. *"Have mercy on me, have mercy on me, O you my friends, for the hand of God has touched me!"* (Job 19:21) Let me go out now. There are few sick and suffering people who have not known the agony of such desires.

Does it seem to you that it is in the choice and ability of your friends to grant your desires? It might strain your body, but it would refresh your spirit and enable you to carry on, on your weary way, rejoicing. These thoughts are bitter drops in your cup of sorrow. There is no harm in your saying, *"My Father, if it be possible, let this cup pass from me; nevertheless, not as I will, but as you will."* (Matthew 26:39). He can take it away and He will if He sees that it will be good for you. But if you find that the cup is still held to your lips, then drink it and learn to say, *"Thy will be done"*. Without this submission, you never will be contented.

Do not imagine that because this spring you have been only a little tempted, that it is a sure sign of increased submission and that you will never be tempted again. The first snowdrop, the first bud, may tempt you again. Or you may pass safely through spring and summer, and then a desperate longing to see the harvest time may fill you.

There may be no harvest field within reach. You feel each day that your desire is unsatisfied, the fulfilment of which would have given you a start back into life and health.

You may feel at any time of the year that if you could only be taken to the seaside, you would get well. Going to the sea, may be impossible. Circumstances may make it so or your doctor may forbid it.

Lie still then and remember that there is a Friend to whom *"the secrets of all hearts are opened, and from whom no desire is hidden[22]"*. He sees your desire. He will fulfil it, if it is for your real good, *"for He is the ruler and governor"*. His never-failing Providence orders all things, in heaven and earth.

Ask God to take away from you all hurtful things, whether they are thoughts, desires or impulses, and to give you those things which are for your good. He will surely do this for you since He is the "Lord of all power and might[23]". Only do not expect Him to fulfil your desires in precisely the way you think would be best. Leave it all to Him who says, *"Be still, and know that I am God"* (Psalms 46:10).

2.6 Circumstances

Do not seek to choose or to change your circumstances. They are the best, the very best for you. *"The only wise God"* (1 Timothy 1:17 AV) has chosen them for you in true love. For *"You have seen the purpose of the Lord, how the Lord is compassionate and merciful"* (James 5:11). Do not seek to change the characters of those about you because you are set in the midst of them for your discipline and correction.

It is not by accident that these particular people are brought into contact with you. Your Father placed them there. Their foibles, deficiencies and mistakes are all for your spiritual growth. They are meant to supply the discipline which is gained while moving in society, by those in health. Many of the things which test us are meant by Him kindly. At any rate try to believe this and receive each thing as kindness, unless there is plain proof to the contrary.

Is it the will of your heavenly Father that you should be shut up in a town when your whole heart revels in country enjoy-

---

[22] from The Book of Common Prayer 1662

[23] from a Collect.

ments? Does the feeling of the deprivation seem to deepen each day, instead of making you become used to it?

Are you tempted to look upon it as wholly stopping your recovery? Does the endless noise seem to stir up all the impatience and restlessness in you? Does it seem to come between your very soul and God?

Do your eyes rest for ever on the same dark, dead houses? Do you long to see green trees and fields once more? Does your heart long for stillness and feel, mournfully, that these blessings are too far away?

But ask yourself who placed you in this city or town. Do you answer "Circumstances"? But who rules "circumstances"? Who could, in one hour, ordain your lot to be in the countryside and let it continue there?

God placed you in this city, or town. God knows all your circumstances, for He placed you in them. He sees them in the minutest detail. He pities you most tenderly with His *"great and endless pity"* but He *"will not spare for the crying"* (Proverbs 19:18 AV) of the child.

If any other lot in life were equally good for you; if any other discipline would have taught you as much of the evil in your own heart or of the Love of God, be assured that He would have "given you the lighter, and kept back the heavier".

Do not dispute with the tempter. Do not let him persuade you that these are bad' circumstances, unsuited to you. Reply immediately and at once, *"Get behind me, Satan! For you are not setting your mind on the things of God, but on the things of man"* (Mark 8:33).

Say: "God placed me here. It is the will of God" and "God is Love" (1 John 4:8). "I know that this is the very best place for me for I was placed here by the only wise God". There is no other answer to all these questionings, temptations, and suggestions. The same answer will serve for every lot in life, for every trial. To wise hearts this certain hope is given: *"No mist that men may make shall hide the eye of Heaven"*[24].

Always try to judge your friends by their circumstances and not by your own. Try to look at things from their point of view and this will prevent you from thinking them unkind or lacking in sympathy. Do not call them 'selfish' because they cannot see into your circumstances and feel the pain and trial that there is in them.

Many things which you would enjoy as a little variety to your life are to others merely ordinary matters in the general run of things or may even be irritations. In the latter case, in kindness they might be trying to prevent you from having any share in them. In the former, they form too much a part of their daily life for them to be conscious that you do not see them in a similar manner.

A move, perhaps from your bed to the sofa, is for you, a great thing. How can you expect sympathy for it? A journey is a matter of great suffering in prospect, at the time, and afterwards. But how can they understand your feelings, those who can move from place to place as they wish?

Ask yourself, did you know how much these things tested the patience of others before you were subjected to them? So how can your friends know about your trials? These are simply instances of ignorance.

Do not then refer to them as lack of love. Friends have the refreshment of air and exercise, meeting with the family at meals, and at other times. They take these things (as you did once) as common mercies, things not to be noticed.

---

[24]This is quotation not attributed in the original book is possibly from memory. It is remembered from the poem, "The Cloud's Silver Lining" p155 of "The Christian Year - Thoughts in Verse" by John Keble, published by Rivingtons (1827). It is likely to have been in the author's own shelf. It can be viewed at http://www.archive.org/stream/a636224902kebluoft. The actual verse should read: "No mist that men may *raise,* can hide the eye of Heaven".

Sickness: its Trials and Blessings

They do not sense the real effect for good which they are having upon them.

They cannot know, therefore, what the deprivation is to you, or what a fight you must maintain in order not to become depressed and indifferent to everyone around. Neither can they know those innumerable frustrations which so greatly distress you. For example the inability to follow what people are saying, the effort to say anything, however necessary it may be, the inability to communicate when you want to speak to them and so many other little burdens that must be shouldered which could be got rid of at once by speaking of them and by having the advice and aid of others.

Perhaps, when family and friends do come, you have forgotten what you wanted to say to them? Or once you begin to speak, they are called away, or remember something that they must do. They promise to return and either are stopped or forget to do so. You, meanwhile, are waiting in expectation, perhaps in impatience.

> Never forget that all your circumstances, even the minutest details, are in the hands of God. Look at them only in this way and not on each circumstance as an accident which may be removed. Receive it as your present lot, as the expression of the will of God towards you. Then you will find that as it is His 'yoke' and bear it in His name and for His sake.

Sonnet[25]

Thou cam'st not to thy place by accident,
It is the very place God meant for thee;

---

[25]This Sonnet is not attributed in the original book but it is by poet and minister, Richard Trench (1807 –1886). He became Dean of Westminster in 1856, and later an Anglican Archbishop.

Sickness: its Trials and Blessings

And should'st thou there small scope for action see,
Do not, for this, give room for discontent.
Nor let the time thou owest to God be spent
In idly dreaming how thou mightest be,
In what concerns thy spiritual life, more free
From outward hindrance, or impediment:
For presently this hindrance thou shalt find
That without which, all goodness were a task
So slight, that virtue never could grow strong:
And wouldst thou do one duty to His mind,
The Imposer's – over-burden'd thou shalt ask,
And own thy need of grace to help, ere long.

2.7 What Effort to make and how to achieve self control

Something very difficult for sick people to decide is what they ought to do? What effort should I make, they ask?

They dread the physical and spiritual effects of overdoing things, more than any mere bodily pain. They know that with every fresh exertion exhaustion increases, the suffering of which, no words can describe. It is not only suffering of body, but also suffering of the soul. It is exhaustion hindering you from prayer until the inner spiritual light grows dim. It is the nervousness causing you such irritability that your day is spent in struggle and fear, in case you should grieve your Lord and Master.

Then there is the incapability to undertake common duties, making you fear that you are sinfully lazy or self-indulgent. There is then the lack of inner peace coming from this; the fear that others will misunderstand you and think you are indeed lazy, which is great suffering. You see the endless length of your future life of pain and weariness and the greatness of your sins. You fear that your spiritual growth has been only backwards and not forward and you are burdened by the intense feeling of lack of sympathy, in those around you.

Sometimes, your own lovelessness actually takes the shape of disliking someone, which is one of the most trying of all the effects of exhaustion. The deep depression and weakness is even influencing your voice and making you seem unkind, when you are not unkind at heart. But the impression that you are, often actually produces the reality.

These are some of the trials which result from an effort made under the weight of great weakness. Then too, there is that exceeding misery of what may be called the pain of malaise, when every bone seems out of joint and every nerve unstrung.

The burden of weakness which you are bearing makes it seem to you that all cares and troubles are focused on you and that all life must be carried in this very moment of unutterable incapacity. You feel that you shall never come out of this spotlight and that seems, in itself, a wearisome weight.

To raise yourself out of this state, by yourself, seems impossible and to take interest in anything or any person almost impossible. All you care for is to be left alone, not spoken to and to be able to feel for a short time that you have no burdens or responsibilities, nothing that you must think about.

Sometimes, however, you are forced to struggle on. There is really no help for, or escape from it, but even then, if you can get but only a quarter of an hour, or even ten minutes alone, the best remedy is to lie perfectly still, on your back and your head as little raised as you can comfortably bear,

with y...
ing at al...

Do not ma...
leg or to sp...
pleasant or pa...
fer themselves t...
you will feel and
trying and you wil...
habit of not thinking...
cipline for you and will...
attempts at acquiring self-...

Try this exercise several time...
for strength and in some of th... . If
possible, never so over-exert yo... ...to the
wretched state described above. ... ...n you begin to feel that it is coming on, unle... ...te impossible,
lie down and be still.

But wait, we have not answered the question yet! What are you to do? What effort ought you to make in any situation? What rules can you follow? You feel that your judgement is so impaired that you cannot decide how much to do, or what is right for you and yet that you are in continual fear of self-indulgence.

Your friends, in their well intended kindness, leave everything to you to judge, as to what you *can* do, what you *will* do, and what you would *like to* do. But you alone know how many things you should *like* to do, which you can never hope to do again, here upon earth.

As to what you *will* do, you wish to have no will, but only to do those things which are *"lawful and right"* (Ezekial 18:5). To be told what to do would be your greatest comfort and delight. Then, as to what you *can* do, you feel quite unable to say and wish that someone could tell you that too.

...at allowance for people
...ness that they either abstain
...n you beyond your power. In the
...y fear pushing you to the point of pain;
...y fear you are falling into a state of invalid-
...would be very distressing to you.

...refore, you must not feel annoyed with them, but keep in mind their intended kindness. It is quite impossible, in many instances for anyone to say what you are able to do. There are certain physical conditions in which doctors can say, to some extent what ought to be possible and what ought not to be attempted. Simple obedience is all that is required. But there are many medical conditions in which it must be left to the person themselves to decide.

Perhaps the following suggestions may be of some assistance, in such cases:

1. First, tell your whole situation to your heavenly Father and ask Him to show you what He would have you do, to reveal it to you, from day to day, hour by hour. Ask Him to teach you to wait upon Him, ask that you may know His will and receive the grace to do it.

2. Do not make plans and rules which you feel are above your strength, but instead do what you feel able to do. If later, you find that you have over estimated your strength, then only do a percentage of it. Nevertheless, some plan or rule will be very helpful to you and lessen your perplexity.

3. Do not let any plan become absolute, but either make it more flexible, or make it more rigid, according to your strength and circumstances.

4. Be at peace with yourself, by constant prayer and self-examination that you are really doing what you can and employing your powers as far as they will go, without too much strain.

Sickness: its Trials and Blessings

5. When you have done all this, do not be agitated, worried or made angry by friends, or even by doctors who tell you that you are merely nervous, or that you could do more, if you try and that you give in too soon, or you are self-indulgent. At the same time, try to determine whether there may not still be some truth in what they say. Do not avoid examining whether something is true. Bear it as "unto the Lord". In silence, submit your will and say in this trial too, "It is the will of God."

6. Do not expect to be able to do exactly the same one day as another and do not make any undue effort to do so. Take the trial of seeming idleness as your lot when it has to be; be thankful when another portion of "work" is given and you are able to do it.

7. Do not expect to do things as well, or as quickly, or as pleasantly as in your days of health. You must learn now, as never before what God says to us: *"My son, beware of anything beyond these. Of making many books there is no end and much study is a weariness of the flesh"* (Ecclesiastes 12:12).

8. After you have done what seemed to you at the time the right thing, be content. Do not question whether it was right, or how far it was right, or whether you should have done otherwise.

You will do well occasionally, to make some attempt to do something new, through a fresh exertion, partly, for the sake of proving that you are capable of doing more than you have been doing, and partly to show your friends that you are wishing to extend your strength, to join in with the family and to employ yourself, as far as possible.

This will often end in bitter disappointment and discouragement. You will find yourself saying, "I tried to step into life again and I could not. I have stepped further than I could go and I am 'destroyed' by weakness again. I seem further off from health than ever and as if I could not get even as far as I did, the next time I try".

Well, this is a dreadful test! But at least it is good to have tried and learned what you can do, and especially that you are not lazy and self-indulgent in doing no more than you had previously done.

What these "efforts" are differ in each case. For some, it may be seeing more friends; to others, writing a letter; to others, being dressed and laid on a sofa near the bed; to others, being taken out of the room; to others, sitting up in a chair; to others, going downstairs; to others, taking a drive, a walk, a journey. Each is according to the various measures of weakness, or ability.

Accept it in your heart that the kindest of friends will rarely fully understand your state and that they may seem to do so today, and tomorrow may seem very obtuse about it. There is only One Person who can fully understand it and who can truly direct you what to do at all times.

Doubtless, you often feel distressed because you are so deeply aware of the pain which each 'act of life' costs you: or, at any rate, the pain which you suffer from it and during it. It seems to you sinfully ungrateful to One who is always helping and upholding you to feel the pain so much more than you feel His ever present almighty aid.

But do not be discouraged. You must not complain about it. You cannot help feeling the pain and suffering. You can have a grateful, thankful heart in spite of it, and be very conscious of His presence and help.

2.8 Irritable Nerves

That large class of diseases called neurological disorders are pre-eminently hard to endure. That class is greatly increased by the limited knowledge that doctors have of the mind and of the workings of the nervous system, and of the real suffering they can cause.

Many peculiarly distressing feelings, which cannot be called 'pain' are known by the name of 'neurological symptoms'. There are few who would not rather hear that certain symptoms are owing to anything, however mortal the disease, than that they are caused by the nervous system. How the word dies upon the heart or rather, how it distresses every part of the mind with suffering.

"Only the nervous system?" What can be said that is more hopeless? What does it mean? Often it means that the symptom or pain is simply not understood and that the doctor can identify no physical cause. Since he must give it a name, he calls it 'nervous'.

The sting of it lies in the words having a double meaning. Used by some, they are meant to express intense suffering. Used by others, they mean 'figments of a diseased imagination', almost self-imposed suffering. These words, said by someone who really feels for you may be repeated to another person and in the passing between them change their meaning. Soon you may hear, "Why are you lying there? Why do you not try to do this or that? The doctor says that your disease is only nervous. Why not break through it then and be like other people?"

How often are you tempted to :

> "Pray for sharpest throbs of pain,
> To ease you from doubt's galling chain?" [26]

All temptations seem on the attack and the tempter ever at hand. You imagine that all the wretched, miserable sensations within you are seen by others. The strange inconsisten-

---

[26]This quotation is unattributed in the original book but the lines are taken from a poem by John Keble for the Second Sunday after Christmas in "The Christian Year". See http://www.lectionarycentral.com/epiphany6/Keblepoem.html for the full text.

cies of mental distress are some of its bitterest trials. You think, at the same time, that everyone can see your trials and fears and also that no one sees it, no one knows it, understands it or cares for it. You think that no one in the world suffers as you do, that your sufferings are quite peculiar, and therefore, cannot be understood.

Do not for one moment try to delude yourself into thinking that this is not a very severe trial. Do not speak of it lightly or make it appear to others that you do not feel it deeply.

Face it all, look this trial full in the face and then say: "Who sent me this trial?" The only wise God. "Why did He send it?" Because He saw that it was necessary for me, perfectly fitted for all my needs, and indeed, the only thing that was. *"And you shall remember the whole way that the Lord your God has led you these forty years in the wilderness, that He might humble you, testing you to know what was in your heart, whether you would keep his commandments or not."* (Deuteronomy 8:2).

You may want to ask Him, "Must I bear this always, for the rest of my life?". But only think about the present, which is all you have. *"Therefore do not be anxious about tomorrow, for tomorrow will be anxious for itself. Sufficient for the day is its own trouble"* (Matthew 6:34). You think about enduring it and bearing it alone. Well, do not! It is God's "visitation". He sees you, and understands you and He made you. He knows what is in you, all your own peculiar feelings, thoughts, character, likings, strength and weaknesses.

He sees you in your day of rejoicing and in your day of sorrow. He sympathizes with your hopes and temptations. He is interested Himself in all your anxieties and remembrances, in all the risings and falling of your spirit. He has numbered the very hairs of your head and the cubits of your height. He compasses you round and bears you in His arms. He takes you up and sets you down. He notes the expression on your face, whether smiling, or in tears, whether healthy or pale.

Sickness: its Trials and Blessings

He looks tenderly upon your hands and feet. He sees your voice and hears the beating of your heart and breathing.

You do not love yourself better than He loves you. You cannot recoil from pain more than He dislikes you having to bear it. If He puts it upon you, it is as you would put it on yourself if you are wise, for your greater good, afterwards.

Never meet this particular form of suffering, nervous suffering, by pure human reason or in any other way than by saying," It is the will of God."

In nervous suffering, the frequent awareness of appearing irritable, of knowing that others think you are, makes the suffering a hundred times worse.

If you could only feel that no one was watching, the trial would be less. Sometimes, perhaps, someone remarks on it to you. A word criticising you for it comes like a blow to the heart and you writhe and cry out for pain. But people see only what is outward. They hear the irritable tone or irritable word and they see the expression on your face. They do not see the unutterable, awful struggle which is ever going on underneath and which, by the grace of God, is preventing much more evil from coming out. How difficult to repress a longing for escape -*"Oh that you would hide me in Sheol, that you would conceal me until your wrath be past, that you would appoint me a set time, and remember me!"* (Job 14:13).

The issue is being aware of sinning, while even fighting with it and resisting it almost to the point of death. It is this which is such agonizing suffering, the seeming to sin against God and to fight against Him, at the same time.

Do not struggle over it, because it increases suffering fearfully. Just lie still and say, *"Lord, you know everything; you know that I love you."* (John 21:17) or say, *"Lord, have mercy on me; this is a sore trial, help me"* for He knows the heart. *"For the LORD sees not as man sees: man looks on the out-*

ward appearance, but the Lord looks on the heart" (1 Samuel 16:7) and He is Love (1 John 4:8), and *"The Lord is compassionate and merciful"* (James 5:12). Surely then, He is grieved for and with you ; He is *"touched with a feeling of your infirmities"*, *"For we do not have a high priest who is unable to sympathize with our weaknesses, but one who in every respect has been tempted as we are, yet without sin"* (Hebrews 4:15). Jesus Himself bore nervous suffering. How intensely He must have entered into them. Every nerve of His was pierced and wounded, and stretched.

Say instead then, "Saviour of the world, who by Your Cross and precious Blood, redeemed us; save us, and help us, we humbly beseech you, O Lord" (Service for the Visitation of the Sick). "By Your agony and bloody sweat; by Your Cross and Passion; by Your precious death and burial; by Your glorious Resurrection and Ascension; and by the coming of the Holy Spirit, Good Lord, deliver us" (The Litany)". *"Fear not, for I am with you; be not dismayed, for I am your God; I will strengthen you, I will help you, I will uphold you with my righteous right hand"* (Isaiah 41:10).

2.9 Taking Drugs[27]

It is often a point of great difficulty and distress to the sick whether they are right to take opiates[28] (which are paink-

---

[27]Priscilla Maurice was prescribed opiates by her doctor. This was common practice by the medical profession in the 19th century, for the treatment of various maladies. Of course, subsequent medical practice restricted their use. Opiates are related to morphine and are most familiar to us today as addictive substances, often abused. Some of what the author says about drugs is specific to the taking of opiates but much of what she says can be applied to other medical drugs today. To remind us of this fact, the editors have sometimes inserted the words 'prescription drugs' in addition to, or instead of 'opiates'.

[28]Opiates were the equivalent of painkillers today. But unlike painkillers, they are addictive.

Sickness: its Trials and Blessings

illers) of any sort. Their doubts generally arise from two causes:

1. The fear of acquiring so bad a habit, which can scarcely fail to cause a kind of addiction

2. Questionings whether it can be right to subdue the sense of pain, when God Himself has sent the pain. For when Christ Himself endured such extreme suffering He refused to drink, even in the midst of His agonizing thirst.

These reasons are not only very plausible but contain much truth. There can be no question that to get into such a habit could be potentially damaging, and even sinful. But this presupposes that there is no necessity for painkillers. If there are no reasons to take opiates, or prescribed drugs, they are simply an indulgence.

But if a trained doctor considers that opiates are necessary, then the patient has no more right to refuse to take opiates than he has to take any other medicine. The taking of any medicine needlessly and habitually would be a very bad habit to acquire. The nature and measure of all medicines that you take, should be regulated by your doctor and we should take all these things passively from the medical profession, looking to its representatives as a servant of God, sent by Him to relieve us. If we find a drug make us dreamy and drowsy, we should mention it to the doctor. If he says that there is no other course of action, that this this will be its effect on us and also that this remedy is necessary, then we are bound to submit our will to his and take the medicine. We must bear the trial as part of the necessary discipline.

But the patient must exactly learn the quantity of a prescribed drug that he or she is to take, and strictly to keep to it, neither diminishing it or increasing it (if it produces pleasant effects as in the case of opiates). The patient should take it always, simply as a matter of obedience. It is certainly true that God sends pain to us, but the same argument, which would prevent us from taking drugs that make us drowsy, would apply to all remedies and we would refuse to try any of them in case they alleviate our suffering.

There is the argument that our Lord refused all alleviations of His pain but this does not hold good. He drank the whole cup of suffering that He might know it all, and understand it all, to be able to sympathise with us. He refused every alleviation of pain so that He might not escape from tasting one drop of that which any of His servants might afterwards be called to drink.

2.10 Longing for Food

At times you may be very much tempted by longings for certain kinds of food. You may have yearnings for some food and if it cannot be obtained, nothing else will do. At home, or in a strange place, you may want something served in some particular way. Your desires are ignored or misunderstood and you either refuse to eat, or do so with lack of relish or disgust, and with a very discontented mind.

You may complain of the cook's obtuseness, become angry with him or her and perhaps complain about the food to other people. Or you may wish for this food at a certain time of day and you may be kept waiting and then lose your desire for, or your will to eat it. Or when food, however carefully prepared is brought, you may have set your mind on something else and either feel thoroughly discontented or loathe the food altogether.

Or you may want first one thing to eat and then another, until those trying to care for you and your friends find you so hard to please that they are at a loss how to meet your wishes. Or you may want something which you know is out of season or is very expensive. A sudden longing overwhelms you that you must have it and you are restless until it is bought.

Sickness: its Trials and Blessings

All these trials are most trying and humiliating. They remind one of *"the corruptible body"* (Wisdom 9:15), *"our lowly body"* (Philippians 3:21). They are trials to which the best disciplined minds and the most self-denying people are subject but they are certainly not as sharp as for those who have always indulged their appetites and have never made any attempt to curb their desires.

To many patients, it is really important what they eat because it really exacerbates their illness to eat certain things. They find out quickly what helps their condition and eating it becomes a habit in their lives which they scarcely ever need to think about. Of course, every patient will feel it a duty to take a food, either ordered by a Physician, or else which they find agrees with them best.

To some perhaps the following suggestions may be helpful:

1. Think as little as possible about *"what you will eat or what you will drink"* (Matthew 6:25). Take what is brought, thankfully, whether or not you feel like eating it. This, of course, implies that you are in a household where things are brought on your behalf. The difficulty is much greater, when a patient has to provide for him or herself. In this case, it is best to set up a simple a plan for the week's menu ahead[29] rarely departing from it so that the order and food come naturally.

2. Think as little as you can of the food longings which so distress you. When they do come, do not reason with them. Try to distract your thoughts to something else. At any rate, do not dwell on them and speak of them rarely, if at all.

3. Look upon them as a trial, as meant to test you and not as any proof of your sinfulness.

---

[29] I have created a whole section on how to plan for and treat chronic illness with diet at http://fatigue.wikispaces.com/diet_recipes and include the best recipes for a restoration of health.

Fasting

Some sick people have found it helpful in disciplining their longings for foods, to abstain from certain food at stated times. But fasting is wrong during a period when your doctor has ordered you to take all the nourishment that you can and when he has prescribed the quantity and quality of your food. But you can give up many little indulgences or eat less of certain things which, if your health needs it, may easily be made up by taking some less agreeable food. You can easily arrange this, especially if you are in control of ordering your own meals.

Whatever you do, do it silently *"with a good will as to the Lord and not to man"* (Ephesians 6:7) and secretly, so that only He that sees in secret may see it. Let how you eat be a "sacrifice". Do not be at peace unless it is and then offer it up, cheerfully and willingly to Him, who loves *"a cheerful giver"* (2 Corinthians 9:7). As He accepted the widow's mite gladly, because she gave all she had, so He will accept the very little offering that you are able to make.

Whatever you do, let it be done seriously, earnestly, deliberately, perseveringly, not as a sudden and impulsive thing, as well as prayerfully. Consider what you will do, then do it at regular and stated times. This will do you much more good than greater things done irregularly and from impulse. The very regularity, the feeling of being under a rule, is an excellent spiritual discipline. Do not begin on too great a scale and then, thinking that you find no benefit from it, give it up. You probably may not experience any benefit at first, perhaps none for a long time, but persevere. You will find a great blessing another day and *"If it seems slow, wait for it, it will surely come, it will not delay"* (Habakkuk 2:3).

Do not make any great effort at first. Begin with a very little thing, so small that you may think that until you try that you shall not feel it and you will soon find that you do. After a time, you may try something else as well and so on.

Sickness: its Trials and Blessings

Occasionally eat some particular food every day for several days, or longer without any variation.

When you have tried all means of disciplining yourself and the food longings still tease you, say, "I must not be disturbed by this as it is a humbling discipline and it is the will of God".

The Blessing of Social and Communal Meals

Remember that the eating apart from a family offers constant temptations. The blessings of social meals are many and great, greater than we have any idea of until we are deprived of them.

Eating together brings a family together. It gives them stated times of meeting, keeps up relationships, gives all members a chance to hear and see much of family life and each others' interests which they would otherwise miss. Eating together removes the selfishness of the meal. It makes a meal not for one's self alone, but for everyone. It becomes something shared and mutual. Conversation helps to make us forget the food and not to find our chief pleasure in food. People who have all meals alone are tempted to selfishness to concentrate on the quality of the food they are eating and of their own capacity to eat and enjoy it. There are many other temptations too small to mention, but which are nevertheless "trying".

Eating Alone

I must not forget one temptation in illness which is the sadness, loneliness and feeling of isolation of eating solitary meals. This seems almost a contradiction because the sick person seldom feels more alone than at meal-times. But He who gives you the blessing of the food is with you. Receive this mercy from His hands and ask Him to bless it. Then you will feel less alone and isolated. Realising His presence while you are at a meal, you will identify with *"...whether you eat or drink, or whatever you do, do all to the glory of God"* (1 Corinthians 10:31)

2.11 Nights

In the days of health, you looked to a night's sleep to renew your strength, to overcome weariness and to enable you to forget depression. You" *laid down and slept"* (Psalms 103:5), and then woke refreshed, or, if you did not, you felt that something was wrong and that you could not be well.

But now the opposite is true. Often the night is your time of greatest malaise, restlessness and sleeplessness. All your anxieties rise again, clothed in blacker thoughts than in the daylight. Night is full of fears, for yourself and for others, full of your most unloving, saddest, most murmuring and discontented thoughts.

Sometimes you say in the morning, *"If only it were evening and at evening you shall say, If only it were morning! because of the dread that your heart shall feel, and the sights that your eyes shall see"* (Deuteronomy 28:67). Your wearied, worn-out body and spirit seem to prefer anything but what you have. You take some sleeping pill and, at length, you fall into a doze but you are perhaps (partly at least) conscious of what is going on around you and of sounds within earshot.

You soon wake unrested and even more wearied in body, more tempted in mind than before. After a while, you fall asleep but your sleep is full of dreams, often most distressing and startling. You dread the night and say to yourself, *"nights of misery are apportioned to me"* (Job 7:3).

Have you ever thought that your words of complaint carry with them the truest comfort and are "appointed?" They do not come by chance or by accident, since God ordered them for you. He knows how many such sleepless nights you need and He will not give you one more than is necessary. Surely, in that last night of His agony, He experienced an extreme of your suffering. He does not appoint such extreme wrestling as He endured for you and when He sends you the sharpest suffering, so that your *"whole head is sick, and the whole heart faint"* (Isaiah 1:5), even then He is near you, He who, in wonderful pity and condescension, has promised: *"The Lord sustains him on his sickbed; in his illness you restore him to full health"* (Psalms 41:3) You know quite what that expression conveys to your mind. You know all the tossing and restlessness that make your bed of sickness so uneasy and such an uncomfortable place.

You know what it is, especially in the night, to be *"afraid also of what is high, and terrors are in the way"* (Ecclesiastes. 12:5) You know the strange imaginations and visions that your poor weak brain conjures up and how hard it is to convince yourself that they are not frightening realities. You know how, sometimes, panic at being alone seizes you and you rightly feel that you ought not to disturb anyone with your fears.

You know too what it is to lie and hear or know that someone nearby is sleeping and to be tempted to envy him or her, until at last you feel as if you could not bear that he or she should have such comforting sleep and you are deprived of it. This tempts you to wake this person.

Beware how you yield to such a temptation! Never on any excuse wake this person, unless it is truly necessary. If you once yield to such a temptation, it will assail you more strongly next time, until your selfishness gains the upper hand and your conflict with yourself will be extreme.

There is no way of meeting this temptation but by looking at these "wearisome nights" as appointed for you, and saying, "It is the will of God". Think when you can, of His unspeakable nearness to you: *"even the darkness is not dark to you; the night is bright as the day, for darkness is as light with you"* (Psalms 139:12).

Think of His agony that night of agony in the Garden of Gethsemane. Your weariness and weakness cannot be greater than His then? You cannot pray, perhaps continuously or however short your prayer is, however broken a sentence or even a mere groan, and it will reach His ears. At any rate, you may seek to feel that *"His left hand is under my head, and his right hand embraces me!"* (Song of Songs 2:6). Lay yourself then quietly down in His arms and believe that *"The eternal God is your dwelling place, and underneath are the everlasting arms"* (Deuteronomy 33:27). *"You will not fear the terror of the night, nor the arrow that flies by day"* (Psalms 91:5). Then: *"Shall your light break forth like the dawn, and your healing shall spring up speedily; your righteousness shall go before you; the glory of the Lord shall be your rear guard"* (Isaiah 58:8).

It is often a great help during the night to repeat poems or hymns or as much of them as you can remember. Or to recite Psalms other words of Holy Scripture or the Services of the Church. Of course, due to your impaired memory it will be a broken recollection, a verse or a line of one, perhaps, and then another. This does not matter. It is a great help in blocking out unholy and distressing thoughts or fears, through occupying the mind and quietening it and so giving it the best chance of sleep.

At first we seem to remember nothing of Bible verses, but gradually more and more will come to mind of what we have read or learnt in the past and thought we have forgotten. It was only lying dormant ready to be used, in time of need. Those who have the ability to read and whose nights are very feverish or who wake shaken by troubling dreams will find nothing so soothing for their minds or so likely to calm their thoughts and prepare them for sleep, as a reading of one or more Psalms, or part of a Bible reading for the day. The painful impression of the dream will fade and they will find it the reading a means by which the Lord works:

Sickness: its Trials and Blessings

"May the Lord give strength to his people! May the Lord bless his people with peace!" (Psalms 29:11)

2.12 Days

After a wearisome night you begin the day either with 'thin' or feverish energy which is soon exhausted and leaves you wearier than before, or else with a sense of exhaustion and unfitness to begin a new day.

You think, "I have so and so to do, so and so to see but how can I do anything?" It is very difficult to bear this sense of impossibility so do not fix too precisely on what you can do and on what you cannot. Let circumstances decide. Things will not develop exactly as you expect them to. When you look forward to the day, everything seems as if it will come at once, at the same time and you wonder how you will cope. Which person shall you put off coming and who will you see? Will it seem like making yourself too important to put someone off? Had you not better see everyone, say nothing about being weak and then later sink under the strain, if you must?

You say, "What line can I draw? What can I do?". If doctors would only *tell* you that you must not do this or that, then you would find no difficulty in obeying them and you would gratefully follow their directions. When they do give such directions, it is a great relief, making it a simple matter of obedience and removing from you the fear of over-indulging or under-applying yourself when, in fact, you ought to be following our Lord's instructions: *"If anyone would come after me, let him deny himself and take up his cross and follow me"* (Matthew 16:24).

The most difficult part of this trial is uncertainty and perplexity, in not knowing what is expected of you. It is not that you want to escape from suffering or from activity, but that in not knowing how much strength you have to do tasks, you do not know how much to use and whether to use what you have or try to preserve it.

To those who have a strong sense of the need to *"make the best use of the time"* (Colossians 4:5) it is a very great distress not to know how to organise one's time so as to be really useful to oneself and to others. They earnestly desire to give every moment to God and for all their activities to glorify Him and not merely to be for present amusement. They want to work for the lasting good of the Church as well as for "this sick member". How to do this is often very perplexing.

Perhaps the following rules can be of some assistance:

> **1.** Ask God in all things to direct and rule your heart, to order it and to direct your mind to studies which will expand it and so prepare it for future usefulness, if it is His will.
>
> **2.** Choose subjects of interest for which there is a natural aptitude and ability.
>
> **3.** Vary your pursuits. Never to continue even an amusement for too long and listen for the well-known indications of approaching fatigue.
>
> **4.** Allow some of your time to be spent merely mechanically.
>
> **5.** Spend some time in mere recreation, without counting it a waste of time.
>
> **6.** If two kinds of reading are to follow each other, spend at least a few minutes between each kind, merely lying still, without even thinking.
>
> **7.** Allow yourself to spend no time in worrying that you can do so very little, but thank God for each thing that He allows you to do.
>
> **8.** Regulate your time so that you choose the part of the day when you are the strongest for the subjects

which require the most attention (and so on, in order).

9. Do not force these activities on yourself as rules or as if they are rules that must not be broken. Let your lessened or increased illness and other circumstances, make you flexible.

10. Do not upset yourself with the opinions that other people offer of your 'duty' to do more, or of exerting yourself more than you do nor dismiss them completely. Lay them before God. Ask Him who knows your heart and what you really can do in every detail, to show you what you ought to do and to give you the will to do it.

11. Do not waste your time with light reading (gossip magazines or fantasies). Everything which expands the mind, enables it to sympathise more with others and to hold closer communion with God. Light reading is apt to occupy the minds of the weak more than of the strong, to distract their thoughts when they ought to be praying and to haunt their dreams and night visions.

12. As much as possible set some objective for yourself and read with this objective in view. Either turn your reading to some special purpose or fix on some subject to which you will turn your thoughts and studies. This will help remove your sense of being without a purpose which is a feeling which afflicts the sick so much.

Choice of Reading Matter

Generally speaking, works of fiction, and especially novels, are not a good choice of reading matter for the sick. They tend to overpower the mind and to prevent it from thinking of other topics. They haunt it by day as by night, so as at times, to increase illness. They are particularly ill-adapted to people who are suffering from nervousness and great weakness and who have not, therefore, the full command and control of their emotions and minds. To them the story they have read may assume an actual form of truth and life. If it is tragic, they may suffer with the sufferers as they read, until their suffering becomes their own and cannot be laid aside with the book, but produces restlessness, feverishness, anxiety, and terror, both in waking and sleeping hours. Besides, there is another very damaging effect, if the story is of great interest, that there is an intense desire to finish it with great impatience and irritability at any interruption. The strain upon the mind and nerves is strung out too long and perhaps causes an increase of suffering and a loss of self-control, for many days.

Surely sick people should avoid everything which lessens their self-control as they have weakness and pain to continually sap it. What they need is everything which will 'brace' the mind and the nerves. If they can read a little, it is better to read such *"things that do not perish as they are used"* (Colossians 2:22), "but tend to help them forward in the right way which leads unto everlasting life" (Service for the Visitation of the Sick).

Travel guides and travel writing contain interest[30]. They take the reader into new scenes and circumstances, and so draw one's thoughts from oneself and one's usual train of ideas.

Nevertheless, there are states of illness in which the occasional reading of works of fiction may be desirable. In very acute pain, toothache or any similar pains, when the mere object is to forget both oneself and pain, a very interesting story will sometimes accomplish the objective for a time. These rules apply mostly to those who have leisure which they desire to use properly, whenever they have strength to do so.

---

[30]Meditating on relaxing places shown and described in travel brochures (free from travel agents) is therapeutic in illness.

Sickness: its Trials and Blessings

But many of the long term sick are in such circumstances in which they have no leisure. Their daily duties, small as they may seem, take all their strength and when they are not doing these necessary little activities[31], they can do nothing but rest.

For you, clearly your duty is to do the work you set yourself with a willing heart and though it seems, at times, to press the very life out of you and increase your distress, try to be very thankful that you have work given to you to do by God Himself.

Offer all your time, strength and gifts to Him, asking Him each morning to show you hour by hour, what He wills you to do. Ask Him to help you to always remember that with each portion of work, and of suffering, comes the portion of strength needed to fulfil it because, *"...Master, I knew you to be a hard man, reaping where you did not sow, and gathering where you scattered no seed"* (Matthew 25:24).

Each morning, consider quietly what seems to lie ahead of you during the day and commit each thing separately to God, asking Him to teach and guide you, to quieten and to strengthen you. It can be done in a few words, in broken words and sentences, if you have no more mental strength.

Ask Him to teach you His will, to guide and direct all your circumstances, to give wisdom in relationships with each member of the family and with friends. Ask that you may receive whatever news the phone, emails or letters may bring or whatever pain they may cause you, calmly and as the will of your heavenly Father. Ask that in whatever phone conversations you have, or any communications that you write, He may guide and direct you. Ask that whatever unexpected circumstances may arise, He will help you to remember that they are from Him.

---

[31]Our advice is to 'do the minimum' possible, in these circumstances.

Sickness: its Trials and Blessings

Ask for wisdom and sincerity in all your interactions with the people around you, with anyone that you expect to see and anyone who may call unexpectedly. Ask, that if you are particularly weak or weary when they come that you may not show it or even utter exclamations of impatience to whoever ushers them in to see you. Ask that you may get through with patience, meekness and quietness all the demands, as well as the pleasurable events of the day. In them all, offer up your will to God.

The Collect with which the Book of Common Prayer begins, "Almighty God, unto whom all hearts be open," used to be, "unto whom every will speaks". Let your will 'speak' to Him. He will hear it and accept it and judge you, not according to what you cannot do, but according to what you can do. Having done all this, constantly remember all day that He is very near to you, and in every new problem, let your will 'speak' to Him.

Do not yield to the temptation of looking ahead to everything as if everything will happen at once, as if all the events of the day will be crowded into a single hour. Do not forecast ahead but take each thing, as it comes and look on it as the present expression of the will of God concerning you. Then regard the next challenge in the same way. Receive your day, piece by piece, from Him who will remember always when He gives you work to do, that you also need strength with which to do it.

You will find it a great blessing to do everything, as much as possible, at stated hours and to do each thing at the same hour every day. Or, if it is a thing that happens only weekly, do it on the same day of the week and at the same hour. It makes things come naturally and easily, and with far less effort. You know what you have to do and can arrange things accordingly. Moreover, habit makes all things so much easier and less burdensome and prevents the constant considering of what you have to do and what you ought to do next.

Often, when you have almost collapsed in spirit, the thought comes, *"If you have raced with men on foot and they have wearied you, how will you compete with horses?"* (Jeremiah 12:5). Put the thought out of your mind. It is a faithless thought. If you need more strength you will have it, be sure of that. Or the call to greater exertion may never come. You have to focus on the present. Leave the future in His hands, who will be sure to do the best, the very best for you.

2.13 Disappointments and Discouragements

Do not expect to be wholly free from weak or depressed thoughts while a sick body is burdening you and causing you *"to groan, being burdened"* (2 Corinthians 5:4). Friends may tell you that any depression is wrong and that what should happen is this: *"Though our outer self is wasting away, our inner self is being renewed day by day"* (2 Corinthians 4:16). They repeat these true words but they make a mistake in their application for *"unless a grain of wheat falls into the earth and dies, it remains alone; but if it dies, it bears much fruit"* (John 5:24).

"What you sow does not come to life, unless it dies. And what you sow is not the body that is to be, but a bare kernel, perhaps of wheat or of some other grain. But God gives it a body as he has chosen, and to each kind of seed its own body" (1 Corinthians 15:36-38). *"It is sown in dishonour; it is raised in glory. It is sown in weakness; it is raised in power"* (1 Corinthians 15:43). *"My frame was not hidden from you, when I was being made in secret, intricately woven in the depths of the earth. Your eyes saw my unformed substance; in your book were written, every one of them, the days that were formed for me, when as yet there was none of them"* (Psalms 139:15-16).

So it is with the spiritual body. How it is moulded and fashioned is hidden from our sight. We cannot see how this severe 'frost', which seems only to harden the ground for now, and even prevent it from receiving the dew of heaven, can be of any benefit for us. But wait, and the spring time will come, when *"The flowers appear on the earth, the time of singing has come, and the voice of the turtle dove is heard in our land"* (Song of Songs 2:12). Then we shall see how necessary the severe frost on the land has been and how it preserved the precious seed.

Do not doubt that *"the inward man is renewed,"* but *"the secret of the Lord is with them that fear Him"* (Psalms 25:14). He knows the inward soul and knows how it is created. So do not be downhearted when your friends offer you deep discouragement. Just say: *"Have mercy on me, have mercy on me, O you, my friends, for the hand of God has touched me!"* (Job 19:21). *"Why are you cast down, O my soul, and why are you in turmoil within me? Hope in God; for I shall again praise him, my salvation and my God"* (Psalms 42:11). *"Though he slay me, I will hope in him; yet I will argue my ways to his face"* (Job 13:15). Do not afterwards return in doubt to this question, or until it ends up with you saying: *"It is hopeless"* (Jeremiah 2:25).

Simply tell everything to "Our Father," or rather say that you cannot tell Him but that He knows your trouble already. Ask Him, if it will please Him, to help you to *"let your light shine before others, so that they may see your good works and give glory to your Father who is in heaven"* (Matthew 5:16). If it cannot be done in the way you hope for, then to help you to say, *"Your will be done"* (Matthew 26:42).

Friends may say that you have "so much leisure time" and that they envy you your leisure. They may say that they sometimes long to be ill so that they may have more uninterrupted time to serve God. They think that illness is such a time for communion with God and for growing in grace. Do not be discouraged by all this. Do not imagine because you do not find these things to be wholly true, that you are in a wrong state of mind and that all the past growth in illness has been only a delusion.

It is 'afterwards' that illness *"yields the peaceful fruit of righteousness to those who have been trained by it"* (Hebrews 12:11).

Leave it all to His righteous judgement and leave yourself in His hands. He knows your situation, your pain, and everything that happens to you and He will judge you according to those circumstances, not according to your estimate of yourself, or of them. *"Therefore let those who suffer according to God's will, entrust their souls to a faithful Creator, while doing good."* (1 Peter 4:19).

2.14 Worries about lack of money in Illness

One more thing must be mentioned as a fruitful source of trial. It can be a blessing, if it is not a source of discontent as well.

Shortage of money is always hard to bear but when sickness is added, it is such a hard a trial, that only He who bore it all, who *"humbled Himself"* (Philippians 2:8), *"took on Him the form of a servant"* (Philippians 2:7) *"had nowhere to lay His head"* (Matthew 8:20) and who passed through the extreme of hunger and thirst for our sakes, can fully understand it or know its hardships. This state is full of temptations of self-pity, anxiety and suffering. But Jesus knows about it all. He not only tasted it, but drank the whole cup, to the very dregs.

Jesus knows how very difficult it is for you to procure the basic necessities of your life, how many things which seem to others essential you must give up. He sees how often you need to eat food which you can scarcely swallow, because you can neither eat nor afford anything else. He sees how often you can eat nothing at all, but instead suffer hunger. He knows the pain of hunger. He bore it for you that He might understand it all and be able to bear you up under the

Sickness: its Trials and Blessings

trial. If your *"strength is famished"* (Job 18:12), He knows it and He pities you.

This level of poverty may not be your main trial. You may not have been tested in this condition, but you are living in constant anxiety and distress, feeling deeply the heavy burdens and expenses sickness causes and that you have no means of meeting them.

Perhaps you have been completely 'laid aside' from the work or calling by which you obtained your 'daily bread'? If you have any relations depending on you, you will feel this, even more deeply. Or, if for the time being, you are obliged to depend on them and know with what difficulty they can meet the necessity, you deny yourself in every possible way. Nevertheless the costs exceed your means and you are sick at heart.

Constant anxiety about money preys on your health, nerves, and spirits. It leaves you less and less probability of returning to work. You think that if you could only afford some treatment or see a particular, private doctor, you would recover. But you feel that you have no money for it.

Then, perhaps this difficulty of finances is removed. One doctor's generosity makes some treatment easy for you, but you have benefited little from it. He orders remedies but those remedies seem to you either out of your reach or to involve great sacrifices. He tells you that you need rest and freedom from anxiety. But he might as well have ordered you to go to China!

You think that if you could only go and live in a sunnier country or by the sea, you would recover, but it is all beyond your income. You need a nurse or convalescent carer but you cannot have one. You are told to take exercise, but you cannot walk and nor can you afford a suitable wheelchair. You are supposed to eat well, which for you is all but impossible and you also feel that you ought to deny yourself every little comfort.

Sickness: its Trials and Blessings

In this way, you become more and more hopeless. All this and the innumerable trials which belong to this state of illness, are best known to those sufferers into whose souls the iron enters[32]. They are indeed bitter griefs[33].

Painful as it may be to you, perhaps it is your duty to make an appeal to friends who are acquainted with your situation, who could help you? Do not let pride keep you from asking for financial help. If our Lord has called you to walk with Him in poverty, remember that He has sanctified the state. Poverty is henceforth "a holy state". Do not let the fear of troubling them hinder you from speaking to them. He has said that He will look on all their acts of mercy as done to Himself: *"Truly, I say to you, as you did it to one of the least of these my brothers, you did it to me"* (Matthew 25:40).

Do not defraud your friends of the blessing which is promised to those who give even *"a cup of cold water because he is a disciple"* (Matthew 10:42)[34]. You will want also to take their rejection humbly and thankfully if they refuse and receive this trial too, as from the hands of God. After all, your true and sure comfort will be that God has called you into this state that He who has passed through it all, who is also our sympathizing High Priest, knows every step of the way.

The Lord Jesus Christ knows all its thorns, snares, and pitfalls, all its crosses and its extreme bitterness. He would not have called you into this suffering, if He had not seen it as being necessary for you.

So do not reason about it. Do not say "Sickness would be easy to bear without financial worries". Only say: *"It is the Lord. Let Him do what seems good to him"* (1 Samuel 3:18). Say "I came into these circumstances by no choice of my

---

[32]Refers to the ancient practice of torturing with iron instruments.

[33]The term 'bitter grief' is Biblical. See Proverbs 17:25 which expresses a mother's sad disappointment at a 'foolish' i.e. a rebellious son.

[34]People in chronic illness can fall through the so-called "safety net" of society

own. It was His will and it is His will that keeps me in them". Be sure that He who fed Elijah by ravens would not suffer you to be *"tempted beyond your ability"* (1 Corinthians 10:13) for "The Almighty God is the Lord of life, and of death, and of all things to them pertaining" (Service for the Visitation of the Sick).

God can raise up friends for you and He will do so, when, and as, He sees best for you. For *"The silver is mine, and the gold is mine, declares the Lord of Hosts"* (Haggai 2:8). Only set before Him all your needs, desires and circumstances, every little trial and even those which are too small to tell to your friends. Answer every sad thought, every suggestion of discouragement, anxiety, fear of the future with, "I must have no worries about the future: it is not in my hands. I have only to think about the present moment for God has placed me in these very circumstances so I must not analyse them in detail. I know that they are the very best for me, because the God of Love has placed me in them. It is the will of God."

2.15 Difficulty in Prayer

Difficulty in prayer is often a subject of pain and trial to the sick. They think prayer should be a blessing but the body and mind are so closely connected that the weakened and suffering body prevents the free exercise of the mind; *"The spirit indeed is willing, but the flesh is weak"* (Matthew 26:41).

You try to fix your thoughts in prayer. You feel that you have so much to ask, so much to pray for. But then a stupor comes over you. You try to rouse yourself but without success. You suddenly awake and think, "Where am I? Have I fallen asleep even at prayer, even while speaking to God?"

It is not so much that your thoughts sometimes wander as that they have 'evaporated' as if they did not belong to you and you have no control over them. Sometimes floating images or figures flit around you.

If you want to pray for your friends, it seems that you can only mention their names before God and cannot ask those things which are requisite and necessary for their bodies as well as for their souls. You rarely, if ever, *"pour out your heart before Him"* (Psalms 62:8). Sometimes you feel that if you could do that, if you could only ask for the strength which you so greatly need, then you know that, *"He would rend the Heavens and come down"* (Isaiah 44:1) and *"He is able to do far more abundantly than all that we ask or think, according to the power at work within us"* (Ephesians 3:20). But it seems as if the very endeavour to pray, breaks up your thoughts. You have no sense of His presence and, which seems worse, no earnest desire to sense it.

Does everything seem to you unreal and an abstraction? Does the eye of your soul seem to be 'dimmed'? Do you almost envy the man in the gospel who said, *"I see men as trees walking?"* (Mark 8:24) since you seem to see nothing. If you catch sight of something, whilst you look, it disappears into the maze of your thoughts. You used to be distressed by wandering thoughts in prayer but now your trial seems to be the absence of all thought.

You feel as if your mind is crumbling. You seem to see it crumble, while you watch it. What is happening to you? Is this the entire loss of your mind? No, it is the pervading presence of weakness, which if it ever pleases God to remove and to give you back your strength of body, will also be renewed.

In the meantime, do not struggle, but be still. It is the duty of faith to believe that since nothing is by chance that He *"without whom not a sparrow falls to the ground"* (Matthew 10:29) appoints each accident of your life. He for whom *"the hairs of your head are all numbered"* (Matthew 10:30) knows the throb of your brow, each hard-drawn breath, each shot of pain, each beating of the fevered pulse and each sinking of the aching heart. Receive, then, these trials not all at once, but one by one, as from His all-loving hands. Thank His love for each. Unite each with the sufferings of Jesus Christ in salvation and pray that He will hereby sanctify them to you.

You do not know what He is doing through each aspect of your illness. But, day by day, you will become more and more like Jesus, the ever-blessed Son. Then, in you too, while you do not know it, God will `be glorified,' and 'shall glorify you'.

It may be that you are thinking that prayer is some hard task and heavy duty? You are forgetting that when the body is low in vitality, the mind shares that weakness too, and that: *"And He who searches hearts knows what is the mind of the Spirit, because the Spirit intercedes for the saints according to the will of God"* (Romans 8:27). This is so much the case that He reads your heart, understands it all and knows what you want to say, far better than you know it. In fact, He knows even before you know it yourself.

What God is looking for is the 'posture' of our soul, the renunciation of our will, or rather your will being so united with His that they are no longer two wills but one Will.

He who created you surely knows how you are made. *"For he knows our frame; he remembers that we are dust"* (Psalms 103:14). It does not say "He once knew it" but "He remembers" it. Do not be afraid then. He is *"compassionate and merciful"* (James 5:11). He does not need your words to enable Him to understand your thoughts. In fact, *"no creature is hidden from his sight, but all are naked and exposed to the eyes of him to whom we must give account"* (Hebrews 4:13). Silence and submission are your offerings now and they will be seen as acceptable in His sight as were your prayers in healthier days. Do not think that continuous speaking to God is the only kind of true prayer. *"O Lord, all my longing is before you; my sighing is not hidden from you*" (Psalms 38:9). God looks at your heart. He sees what is in it, things which you cannot frame into words, which you cannot express, but which He fully understands.

You cannot tell God anything. He knows it already. You can only say, *"Lord, help me"* (Matthew 15:25). He sees and will surely answer you. You say when you wake in the morning and in the night, and often in the day, "Vouchsafe, O Lord, to keep me this day without sin"[35]. That is prayer, the truest prayer.

God does not measure a prayer's worth by its length, but by its sincerity. The mere sense of being in His arms, of His understanding you, loving and embracing you, that is prayer because it is the losing yourself in Him.

Do you not often find answers coming into your thoughts? You scarcely thought that needs had been scarcely expressed. But He is very near, yes, in fact within you. You need not speak but He interprets your silence. He saw you and He said for you, *"The spirit indeed is willing, but the flesh is weak"* (Matthew 26:41) and the Holy Spirit *"helps us in our weakness. For we do not know what to pray for as we ought, but the Spirit himself intercedes for us with groaning too deep for words"* (Romans 8:26).

Never mind your inability to speak. Just offer up your whole self saying, "You know what I cannot speak, and why I cannot speak as you know all things."

But when you say, *"I come to do your will, O God"* (Hebrews 10:7, 9) do not be disturbed if the answer is, *"A body have you prepared for me"* (Hebrews 10:5). Do not be dismayed if more suffering is the answer to your submission, if it seems to be a mere conflict between the flesh and the spirit. If so,

---

[35]From the "Te Deum" which is an early hymn of praise. Usually thought to be written by Saint Ambrose and Saint Augustine, some scholars assign it to Nicetas, Bishop of Remesiana (in the 4th/5th century).

it is an honour because it likens you to your Lord and Master, to whom the same answer was given. The lesson for you now is that your *"strength is to sit still"* (Isaiah 30:7).

What if you feel too weak to ask Him anything, too weak to open your heart at all? If this is the case, and you are not deceiving yourself, then in such extreme sickness, it is simply enough to lie still and to trust to God for an answer to what you would have prayed, if you could, but cannot. "He will pour down upon us the abundance of His mercy"[36]. When He has mercy, it will fall on us and we shall be moistened as with the dew. Gradually we shall be bathed in it until it penetrates into every part of us.

No thoughts, fears or sins need make a separation between us and Him or lead us to imagine that because of them, God's grace cannot reach our hearts. He will "forgive us those things whereof our conscience is afraid[37]". He sees our dark thoughts and how they separate us from Him, and from our brothers and sisters and He knows what a fearful trial they are to us. He knows that they come out of weakness and nervousness and about them too, He says: *"The spirit indeed is willing, but the flesh is weak"* (Matthew 26:41). *"In the days of his flesh, Jesus offered up prayers and supplications, with loud cries and tears, to him who was able to save him from death and he was heard because of his reverence. Although he was a son, he learned obedience through what he suffered"* (Hebrews 5:7-8).

You are learning obedience too, so do not refuse the lesson. You may, perhaps, have no exciting or pleasant thoughts in prayer but, you could not hate sin if He had not taught you to do so. Hating what God hates, shows love to Him. You cannot love with your affections, love with your will or 'will yourself to love'. If you cannot love as you would like to, do

---

[36]Collect - Twelfth Sunday after Trinity.

[37]Collect - Twelfth Sunday after Trinity.

Sickness: its Trials and Blessings

what you can. If all love seems to have died within you, cleave to God with your mind and understanding.

If the idea of God seems to your mind, as if it were an idea with no reality, if your prayers seem only words with no substance sent idly into the ether and not ascending to God; if things unseen seem to you are only a dream and things seen, the only reality; if fervent words do not move you, if thoughts of love do not set you on fire, if the passion of Christ does not touch you, do not get depressed. "Out of the deep cry to God" and He will hear your voice[38]

"Though he slay me, I will hope in him; yet I will argue my ways to his face" (Job 13:15). These great and holy words mean yet more: "If He slays me, I will trust in Him,' not *although* only, but *because* He slays me.

It is life to be touched by the hand of God. To be put to death by Him is, through the Cross of Christ, the pledge of Resurrection. May our hearts be strong and renewed when, at his compassionate touch, our 'sinew shrinks?'[39] It is the Redeemer's hand, which upholds, while, at the same time, it seems to cripple. His hand strengthens us while it seems to put forth His strength against our weakness. By His strength we have power with God, while we can only weep and make weak prayers to Him.

Not sensible comforts, nor delight in prayer, nor His very voice to the heart, nor tokens of His presence, nor the overflowing of His consolations, may be such a proof of His love for the soul, as the unseen, unfelt strength by which He keeps the fainting soul alive to trust in Him. People in health have little or no idea of what the state of weakness involves. They like to tell the sick that they must have "so much time

---

[38]"Out of the deep I cry to Thee" is a hymn of Martin Luther (1483-1546).

[39]Sinew is used to make bows. Sinew must be shrunk through drying to become useful for making weapons. This could apply to making "spiritual weapons".

for prayer", that it is their "vocation" and that they are "prayer missionaries".

How the hearts of the sick sink at these words. "So much time for prayer?" Yes, you know that it may seem so, to those who know nothing of the trials of illness. But you also know that sometimes it seems quite impossible to pray at all, and that often the sheer effort required for any continuous act of fixed attention is impossible. You fall into dreamy imaginations, prayers pass into mere thinking or into the entire absence of all thought.

Sometimes your condition keeps you from even realizing God's presence at all. You feel that you are in His presence but as if you were asleep in His arms, unable to think, or meditate, or pray, or realize anything. You are just conscious of this and nothing else. "I am in His arms. He holds me, He is embracing me, surrounding me with His love, with Himself". But then the thought comes, "How ungrateful not to love Him more, not to speak to Him and to *pour out my complaint before him. I tell my trouble before him*" (Psalms 142:2).

The answer is that He knows that you wish this just as He knows all your heart. He knows that it is a grief to you that you cannot do it. *"In the path of your judgements, O Lord, we wait for you. Your name and remembrance are the desires of our soul"* (Isaiah 26:8). He knows that you cannot get beyond that. He will not expect anything of you that you cannot do, for it is His will that you should suffer as you do. He has sent the trial.

In one sense, He expects less of you than you do of yourself. He knows that it would be a pleasure for you to feel that you are in a higher state. But He will bless and sanctify to you the trial of being in a lower state. Therefore, you may *"rest in His love"* (Zephaniah 3:17).

Sickness: its Trials and Blessings

That same peculiar stupor of mind extends to everything so, *"Is it not therefore of the body?"* (1 Corinthians 12:15). Do not attempt continuous acts of prayer when they are impossible. *"They shall lay their hands on their mouths; their ears shall be deaf"* (Micah 7:16). Does not that verse express silence? Let your *"soul be silent upon God"* (Psalms 42:1 AV). In stillness, you will find God. *"And after the earthquake a fire, but the Lord was not in the fire. And after the fire, the sound of a low whisper."* (1 Kings 19:12)

Even when continuous prayer is impossible, it is often a great help to fix on certain topics and to remember each one at some stated time during the day. Try not to do more than remember this topic. Thing of it, keep it in mind, bear it on your heart before God. So though you may not be able to pray for your friends as you want to do, you may remember them in your heart and name them one by one, before your *"Father and your Father, my God and your God"* (John 20:17).

Do not make a great effort to pray. Do not think about how you are not praying, unless your prayers occupy a given time, unless they seem very fervent or you feel delight in them.

"Lord, help me" (Matthew 15:25). *"My Father, this is a time of need: help me now. Graciously look upon our afflictions. Pitifully behold the sorrows of our heart. Forgive all my sin"* (Psalms 25:18). *"O God, make speed to save us. O Lord, make haste to help us"*. *"Jesus, Son of David, have mercy on me!"* (Luke 18:38). *"I am severely afflicted; give me life, O Lord, according to your word!"* (Psalms 119:107). *"Help me. Lord, have mercy upon us. Christ, have mercy upon us"* (Book of Common Prayer).

These sentences, and numerous others, will come to you as need arises and above all, the Lord's Prayer will convey your wants to Him. It will bring you as much peace and blessing as the most lengthened prayer ever did in days of your strength and vigour.

We must remember too that it is not our prayers alone that are offered. For they are all moulded afresh for us, offered again, by our Intercessor Jesus Christ and His intercession has also this further perfection. It is the prayer not only of Divine Love and knowledge, but of perfect human sympathy. *"For we do not have a High Priest who is unable to sympathize with our weaknesses but one who in every respect has been tempted as we are, yet without sin"* (Hebrews 4:15).

What, as God, He could never taste, as Man, Jesus tasted to the dregs. He knows us, but as perfect Man. The mysterious knowledge of personal experience, of personal suffering in human flesh which He gained on earth, He still has in Heaven. Even before the eternal throne, He has still a perfect sense of our infirmities, of all the mystery of human sorrow which He learned on earth, from the manger to the Cross.

It is especially in this connection that St. Paul encouraged us to pray. *"Let us then with confidence draw near to the throne of grace, that we may receive mercy and find grace to help in time of need"* (Hebrews 4:16). Out of this Perfect Love, knowledge, and sympathy, He perpetually intercedes for each of us, according to our trials and our circumstances. Nothing can come upon us which does not have its counterpart and response in His perfect compassion.

While He prays for us, He feels with us. To Him we may go, as to One who is already pleading for us. Through Him, we can approach God as if with His perfect merits which He has given us, for our own. They are ours, because they are His. Because they are His, therefore He has given them to us. Though you cannot pray, The Lord is praying for you. Only put yourself into His hands and let Him plead for you. Give yourself up to Him. If your will is one with His, what He asks will surely be what you would have desired for yourself

Sickness: its Trials and Blessings

if you had had the power to ask or think. For He knows everything.

He knows how bitter it is to you when your friends seem to imagine that your time is spent in prayer and meditation and when they seem to be relying on your prayers to bring down blessings on them. You know that if you tried to explain your situation to them, they would either think that it was your humility that you would not declare your own saintliness, or they would think you in a very bad spiritual state indeed, and almost needing a complete change of heart.

Do not be depressed. *"God Himself is Judge!"* (Psalms 50:6) and *"You know when I sit down and when I rise up; you discern my thoughts from afar. You search out my path and my lying down and are acquainted with all my ways"* (Psalms 139:2-3). You will ask Him, once or more times, if it pleases Him to give you the spirit of *"prayer and of supplication"* (Philippians 4:6).

If still He sees it necessary for your development, to keep it from you, then ask Him to bless the trial or at least to listen to your breathing or your groaning and to give you a sense that He is listening to you, a sense of His presence and His nearness. If, for a time even this blessing is denied, if you cannot feel that He is near, at least try to believe it. If you must say, *"Behold, I go forward, but He is not there, and backward, but I do not perceive Him; on the left hand when He is working, I do not behold Him; He turns to the right hand, but I do not see Him"* (Job 23:8-10). Try to say too, *"But He knows the way that I take: and when He has tried me, I shall come forth as gold"* (Job 23:8-10).

Though you are, indeed, in this hot furnace, the Refiner is sitting nearby, watching you closely. He notices each portion of dross[40] and impurity, as it falls away. You may not see

---
[40] When precious metals are refined, they are heated to a high temperature in a furnace which separates out the impure elements (base metals)

Him, but He is sitting nearby, watching you tenderly and patiently. He *"puts your tears into His bottle"* (Psalms 56:8) even though they are only 'tears of the heart' and never expressed by the eyes. He sees them all, *"and not one of them is forgotten before God"* (Luke 12:6).

Even if you seem to yourself totally forsaken by God, it cannot be worse for you than for Jesus, who said, *"My God, my God, why have you forsaken me?"* (Matthew 27:46) At least, He is with you in the deepest sympathy and with most tender pity. You say, *"O my God, I cry by day, but you do not answer, and by night, but I find no rest"* (Psalms 22:2).

"You have put me in the depths of the pit, in the regions dark and deep. Your wrath lies heavy upon me, and you overwhelm me with all your waves ... Your wrath has swept over me; your dreadful assaults destroy me. They surround me like a flood all day long; they close in on me together" (Psalms 88:6,7,15,16).

But you can never say the words of Christ. You cannot feel *"Look and see if there is any sorrow like my sorrow, which was brought upon me, which the Lord inflicted on the day of his fierce anger"* (Lamentations 1:12) or there is no *"grief like unto my grief"*[41]. For there is One [42]who bore your griefs and carried your sorrows, and who bears them now.

You do not dare to describe your temptations in case you could be suggesting wayward thoughts to some other sufferer in whose mind they have so far found no place. But do not fear to tell them all to Him. No temptation that can assault you can be strange to Him *"because He Himself has suffered when tempted, He is able to help those who are being*

---

which are called 'dross'. This leaves pure silver or pure gold behind in "The Refiner's fire".

[41]From "The Sacrifice" by George Herbert see www.poemhunter.com/pcem/the-sacrifice-2

[42]The burden Christ carries is to bear our grief, in addition to His own (and that of all the redeemed).

Sickness: its Trials and Blessings

tempted" (Hebrews 2:18). In those forty days in the Wilderness, every form of temptation came before Him. Do not fear to lay open everything to Him since the devil tempted Him to throw Himself from a pinnacle of the Temple. He overcame the tempter in order that they who trust in Him might never be overcome, by His own temptations.

Much of the failure to pray in your case, is owing to physical suffering, to extreme exhaustion, to having lost the power of judging justly, of seeing how things truly are. This, perhaps, seems poor consolation and it is better to say you cannot understand yourself. Do not try to understand yourself as you will only get into endless perplexities. So do not reason about mysteries. Do not question yourself about your state before God, but lay it open. Open your heart, open yourself, open your will, before Him. Words are not necessary.

God only wants you to offer yourself and to let Him do with you as He sees best. Sometimes it is a great help to use the prayers of the Church, the Collects, or the Service for the Visitation of the Sick[43]. Do not think it must be read in a formal way or that it is a very formal thing to have set prayers or a Service on purpose to read to the sick when you visit them.

Would the Church have provided for all her members if she had furnished no Service for the Sick? Surely she could not if she were a true mother *not* do so. The more you study the Service for the Visitation of the Sick the more you will find it adapted to your needs.

This Service teaches in a wonderful manner what the trials, temptations, duties, responsibilities and blessings of sickness are. The whole meaning and purpose of sickness is illuminated. Since the Collects are short and the words exactly express the wants of the sick, they are the greatest help to prayer for all those who are willing to use them.

---

[43]The Service for the Visitation of the Sick is published in the Appendix.

2.16 Absence of Work

Sick people are either in such a situation that their work is very demanding but seems far beyond their strength; or else they are laid aside from all work and constantly distressed because they are useless, or so they suppose.

Perhaps you may be able to trace a connection between some part of your trial and past times and find them closely linked together? Have you ever discovered how wonderfully this or that aspect of sickness is like a chastisement for past sins?

If you are now called to work, in the midst of great weakness, weariness and suffering, were there no strong desires for work in the past when it was God's will that you should be idle and quite laid aside. Did you then recognize that state as the will of God, as one to be desired and to give thanks for, because it was His will? Were you restless under that discipline? Did you ever cry out, "Oh if I could only have work! I was never formed for idleness. My deep and earnest desire was work to glorify God, but it is all destroyed, all my dreams are broken. But I have no less desire to do it. I could work so much more purely now than I could or would have done then. Indeed, I have in the past prayed to be *"sanctified completely"* (1 Thessalonians 5:23) but I never expected that He would answer my prayers in this way?"

Was there never a time when such thoughts came to you? Did you never beat against the cage in which the Lord had shut you up, and try to break your way out? Did you never so occupy yourself with complaining that you missed many precious lessons and did not hear His *"still small voice"* (1 Kings 19:12)? Do you not know that this is His own "visitation", His own coming home to you, to talk with you in your own bedroom, where He can find you still?

Sickness: its Trials and Blessings

If, in the past, instead of being still and *"communing in your own heart"* (Psalms 4:4), you were complaining, can you wonder if He said at last that He would grant your request? Perhaps He has answered it just as you asked and has given you work. But now the work seems beyond your strength.

Well, do not complain. He has simply heard your cries for more holiness and work to glorify Him and has shown at once His fatherly correction and forgiveness, by sending you work, and with it, suffering.

God saw that you could not bear the work on its own. It would have made you proud, high-minded and independent. You would never have known yourself or how much you wanted the work to glorify you, for the sake of doing it and for the very love of activity.

He saw it all and said, "You shall have your desire - you shall have work; but with it you must have a constant test of your work and of your motives. If you really wish to serve me, then here is the work which I give you to do. Will you do it for the love which you bear me because you love my service? It will cost you very much suffering, but it is your own choice".

Receive work then now, receive it all, and do not falter from anything. Do not complain but *"Humble yourselves, therefore, under the mighty hand of God so that at the proper time he may exalt you"* (1 Peter 5:6). You are being humbled as chastisement, as punishment, but at the same time give hearty thanks to Almighty God for the work which He gives you to do. Do it before His sight, as *"rendering service with a good will as to the Lord and not to man"* (Ephesians 6:7). Do it cheerfully, thankfully, submissively, humbly and take each little thing as part of it, as the expression of the will of God towards you. Take it patiently, penitentially and silently, offering up your will to God as a *"living sacrifice"* (Romans 12:1).

Sickness: its Trials and Blessings

Be careful how you turn your blessings into burdens. Rejoice that he has made you *"worthy of his calling"* (2 Thessalonians 1:11) and if at the same time He calls you to suffer, believe that you could not do your work properly or as safely, if you had not at the same time received suffering to chasten, humble and subdue you and to make you work all your works, in God.

It is very frustrating to feel day by day so crushed and oppressed, as if the life of your spirit were being pressed out of it. But take care how you complain. Your active spirit would surely feel it a hundred times a greater trial if you were not allowed to work at all but called to lie still.

Beware of complaining and murmuring against God, in case God should *"answer you in your folly"* (Proverbs 22:5) and give you the thing which you have thought you would prefer. Remember that your work comes only moment by moment and just as surely as God calls you to work, He gives the strength to do it.

Do not think in the morning, "How shall I get through the day? I have such-and-such work to do, people to see, and I do not have enough strength for it". No you do not have enough strength, but you do not need it.

Each moment, as you need it, the strength will come. Do not look forward even an hour. Circumstances may be very different from what you expect. You will be carried through each thing *"on eagles' wings"* (Isaiah 40:31). Do not worry yourself in advance but take each thing quietly, as it comes.

Nothing is such a help to anyone, but above all to the sick, as quietness of spirit, self-control and presence of mind. They should be cultivated. We have to regret that we never cultivated these things in our earlier life. It will make the conflict harder now, but *"with God, nothing is impossible"* (Luke 1:37) and He can *"work in us to will and to do of His own good pleasure"* (Philippians 2:13).

Sickness: its Trials and Blessings

Do you sometimes cry out internally, *"Oh, that I had wings like a dove! I would fly away and be at rest"* (Psalms 55:6). Be content. There *"remains a rest"* (Hebrews 4:9) for you, *"an inheritance that is imperishable, undefiled, and unfading, kept in heaven for you"* (1 Peter 1:4). Wait a little while and you shall enter it *"For still the vision awaits its appointed time; it hastens to the end--it will not lie. If it seems slow, wait for it; it will surely come; it will not delay"* (Habbakuk 2:3). In the mean time, remember that *"For we who have believed enter that rest"* (Hebrews 4:3). Let us enter into God. He is our rest, and He says: *"Come to me, all who labour and are heavy laden, and I will give you rest"* (Matthew 11:28). Let us look upon all our burdens as laid upon us by Him, our yoke as His yoke, which is light, because He bears it with and for us and takes off all the heaviest part of the weight from us.

Let us regard all our circumstances as the expression of His will, as His own voice speaking. This will give them a sacred character and be the surest antidote to complaints.

The opposite trial, the absence of all direct employment, no apparent work, is no less trying. It is impossible to say that one state is harder to bear than the other, as it depends entirely on the character, circumstances and habits of the individual. To one, a life of activity, under any circumstances, may be less trying than a life of mere sickness. To another, work or responsibility are such burdens that they would almost prefer to do nothing than be in a state which involved these things.

It is very foolish and sinful in sick people to compare their lots and say, "How much harder mine is to bear than yours! You are quite free of such and such trials, which are to me so very hard to bear. If I had such and such a thing, which you have, I could bear anything. Yours is such a useful life but mine so entirely useless". One person may say, "You have work to do. If I had only that, all the rest would be easy to bear". Another may say, "How I envy you the quiet and rest that is given to you! My cross is having none".

Why should we wonder if this is what happens? *"The heart knows its own bitterness, and no stranger shares its joy"* (Proverbs 14:10). This is knowledge for the heart alone and Him who searches the heart. Yes, each person's deepest grief is hidden from the eyes of his neighbour. Sickness no more makes trials similar, or characters similar, than health does.

If you wanted rest when you had work given you to do, if you sometimes longed for sickness to give you, as you imagined, time and space to serve God, if you often complained that you had no time, groaned under the burden of your work and did not do it with a free and glad heart, then do not be surprised if you have the answer to your cravings (for they were scarcely prayers). You wished for rest and you have it.

Seek to improve this period and season of trial. Do not spend your time in desultory desires for vague blessings but earnestly ask God to *"let me know why you contend against me"* (Job 10:2). Watch to see what He will say to you and what you shall answer when you are reproved (Habbakuk 2:2). There is much for you to do, even in this state.

So lie still and He will be your Teacher. Do not let the voice of discontent or sadness drown out His voice. Ask Him to: *"Apply your heart to instruction and your ear to words of knowledge"* (Proverbs 23:12). Answer all questionings and silence all sad thoughts with : "It is the will of God."

2.17 Anniversaries

There are few who have been chronically ill for a long time who do not have a dread of all anniversaries. The whole character of their life has changed, the 'clouds' seem to have 'gathered' and the bright spots of life are few. Those days and festive seasons which once looked bright and joyous

Sickness: its Trials and Blessings

and welcome, now, when they come round with the seasons again, seem to be *"full of trouble"* (Job 14:1). Anniversaries bring to mind the things that were bright and joyous, but no longer are.

There was the unbroken family then, voices to be heard which are no longer heard[44], except in one's saddened memory. There was precious sympathy to be received, joyful greetings and the sharing of joy. Life looked bright and the glad spirit counted joy on joy. You expected only brighter joys and blessings yet to come. There was no thought of such changes then. But years passed and possibly, friend after friend passed on and their loss made this life sadder and more lonely. Then the sickness came and your life was completely altered. Now the seasons come round again and often they only seem to mock one's sorrow.

Your birthday returns yet again. It used to be a glad day but now you dread it. Why? Perhaps because it tells you that another year has passed, another long year of sickness and you are still here in your room, just the same, no hope of being better, with no brighter things ahead.

Your birthday morning arrives. It saddens you to hear the usual greetings "Many Happy Returns!" Actually, you would prefer no more "returns". You do not accept that they can be "happy". You think, "Why upset me like this? Don't remind me of my birthday. Please let this day go unnoticed".

If you feel this, you are much mistaken. In fact, you would not like it to pass unnoticed. You would find it pure insensitivity if no one noticed it, if no one cared about you. Do not turn it away without love as if you were annoyed. These birthday wishes are meant in true kindness. Receive the greetings heartily, pretend they give you pleasure and then

---

[44]It is hard not to read this chapter without sensing that Priscilla Maurice is thinking of the loss, in the first bloom of youth, of her sister, Emma and of their cousin, all Christian believers of the same kind.

Sickness: its Trials and Blessings

think whether there is any reason why this should be a glad day for you.

Your birthday: what is that? Well, it is the anniversary of the day that you were born into this world of sorrow. Yes! But what is it? Was it not the day in which life began in you, life which shall well up to eternal life? Would you now have the assurance of the blessing of everlasting life, if your life had not begun here on earth? We make a mistake in separating this life from that which is to come. It is all one thing. Life begun here and is carried on into eternity. Therefore you should give thanks for your creation, for your birthday.

Think again what you would be, without this sickness. Would you understand the character of our Lord, *"The man of sorrows"* (Isaiah 53:3) Would you not be so unlike all His people, with whom you hope to live forever?

You should rejoice, then, in this, your time of suffering and welcome every return of the day of your birth, as a day of blessing? Let your birthday be a happy day, a day of thanksgiving for your "creation and preservation, and all the blessings of this life"[45].

Even though you meet your birthday, separated from the family, rejoice in all their loving attempts to unite you with it, and receive their greetings gladly until they become a part of yourself and make you glad.

The anniversary of the birthday or of the departure of one of your dearest earthly treasures comes. It seems to you as a day of pure sadness. How will you face it? If they were here you would not be alone, and your sickness would be cheered. You would have their constant sympathy. They understood you. They knew the sorrows and the loneliness of sickness. They always had words of tenderness and of encouragement for you. But this person has gone. Gone

---
[45]From the Prayer of General Thanksgiving, The Book of Common Prayer

Sickness: its Trials and Blessings

where? Into eternity? Then they are not far from you. You know not how near.

Do not count the dead as 'gone'. It is only their conversation that has ceased. You can hold communion with them even now and you need not be separated from them. Your very sickness may bring you nearer to them because, being cut off from your fellow humans, you can live closer to their holy company and with fewer interruptions.

You can make their anniversaries like holy days, days which draw you nearer to God and to the unseen world. Then, gradually, these days will lose their sadness and have a peaceful character instead.

Seasons, too, are great trials to the sick and the lonely. The New Year comes and brings its own note of sorrow. What has been said of birthdays applies too, to that day.

How can Christmas Day be a happy day for a sick person? Can it be kind to wish them Christmas joys and Christmas blessings? Christmas is that glad time of family meetings which they cannot share. Christmas, the season of festivity. How can it be a happy season to them? Surely, above all seasons it reminds them of departed joys and tells them that the days have arrived in which they say that they *"have no pleasure in them"* (Ecclesiastes 12:1).

Yet there are two ways of enjoying Christmas which all sick people can share in. One is to enjoy it for and with others, to be happy because others are happy; *"Rejoice with those who rejoice, weep with those who weep"* (Romans 12:15) and to make their pleasure your own. Enjoy the family meeting for, and with others, because they are enjoying it, to lose oneself in them.

The other way is, to remember what Christmas is: it is the celebration of the birthday of our Lord and Saviour Jesus Christ. The day on which He came into this world and became *"acquainted with grief"* (Isaiah 53:3 AV). The day on

Sickness: its Trials and Blessings

which He began to take upon Him weakness, suffering, feebleness and helplessness, on which *"He took our illnesses and bore our diseases"* (Matthew 8:17). Christmas is the time when He began to know what loneliness, lack of sympathy and being misunderstood by others really meant. The day on which He came to redeem us from sin, to take away the curse, that curse which involves sickness.

Surely Christmas Day is a day on which sick people *should* rejoice and be glad. They should welcome Christmas as a joyful day. If they cannot go to church and worship with others, should they not be more independent of the need for church worship on this, than on any other day, because the thoughts which they need are stimulated by what is going on around them, by the decorations in their room, by Christmas greetings, by the festivities around? Let us then be glad and rejoice and keep a "Happy Christmas".

For some, Lent is a very unhappy season. They cannot go to church nor can make an outward penance although it is a time of humiliation. They say that perhaps they ought to do something and yet what can they do? The whole season of Lent is a weight and a burden to them, a time of sadness.

It is best generally not to attempt much abstinence during Lent and not to be anxious because you can do so little. You may find some small thing to do, enough to keep you mindful of the season. It may be some little abstinence, which of course you will consider it your duty not to allow to interfere with the progress of your recovery.

Let it be something which will neither do you any harm, or weaken you. It could be some little good work done regularly. It may be some little self-denial. Each person must judge according to circumstances.

A season of humiliation is especially one which should come home to your heart, not as one of sadness, but as a mirror of your own situation, suited to remind you of the meaning of sickness and its humiliation. This season ends and passes into one of joy and thanksgiving.

Have you no part in Easter? Is it too "glad" for you? Surely *Easter* means much more to you? Passion-Week speaks to you of His death which has redeemed death for you, and "opened the kingdom of Heaven to all believers[46]". The glorious assurance of your own resurrection follows this Holy Week. Jesus rose from the dead as a sure token that we shall, if we "*are found in Him*" (Philippians 3:9) rise too. Let us rejoice and give thanks and rise out of the 'grave' of all our sadness, be "*seated us with him in the heavenly places in Christ Jesus*" (Ephesians 2:6). We can pass through it refreshed and thankful, hoping that when a few more Easters have passed, we shall have finished our days of suffering and shall "rise with Him to life eternal"[47].

On Ascension-Day, Whit-Sunday and all the Feast Days of the Church, we find fresh reasons for rejoicing and go from step to step, rising higher above the darkness and sorrow of life, finding joy, or at any rate no painful sadness in each anniversary, whether it belongs to our own individual life, or to that of the universal Church.

2.18 Family and Friends

In this life, pleasures and pains are so closely connected, that often the things which bring the greatest enjoyment are also the most 'fruitful' sources of trial.

Although we derive our greatest earthly happiness from the kindness and love of our family and friends, they can cause us the most trial. Their visits are often a great discontent and disappointment to the sick. People may be in a hurry and before you have overcome the excitement of seeing them, they have left. Or they may come at just the time

---

[46]From the "Te Deum" (see also footnote 30)

[47]See references in John 5: 28-29

when you feel least able to enjoy their visit when you were very weak, or more than usually ill. Or your friends may seem absent-minded and you may think them cold and unkind, lacking in sympathy, uncaring for your circumstances.

Or their conversation may be very lacking in interest or they may have touched on great range of subjects and yet elaborated on none? The outcome is that you feel wearied and dissatisfied. You know that nothing is more exhausting than this kind of visit, especially if the talk has been too much about people, or mere passing events, or gossip.

Or, your friends may have stayed with you much longer than you had strength for, though at the start you really enjoyed their company. Finally, you become so weary that you lose your pleasure in the visit if not in them.

In their kindness they may have urged you to make an effort which you know is impossible and you may think that they do not understand you and feel almost angry with them. You part with them with an estranged feeling, which, if it is not resisted, increases. Or you may feel constrained in your conversation or that, with almost every visitor, there is some subject to be avoided, so that all frank discussion is prevented.

But surely this is a trial which belongs to those in health as much as to you? Those in health come more into collision with others and suffer from this trial more than you do. But you are "laid aside" so that you have time to think about things, see things separately from others. Therefore, it seems to you as if your lot is a very trying and isolated one.

The subject of seeing people is a very difficult one for the sick. Some are quite exhausted by the many people they see. It is an incessant burden upon their resources, a distraction to their minds and takes up the best of their time. To some this is a great enjoyment. They enjoy the wearing 'thin' of their energies in this way.

Sickness: its Trials and Blessings

To others seeing too many people comes in the form of real, constant trial, a daily cross. If they could choose to see only certain people, and at certain times, they would indeed feel thankful for it. But if circumstances make it plain that this is their "calling", they have no right to try to alter it, or to complain about it. They should learn how to welcome each person as the present message sent to them by God, for their profit, either to help or bless them, or to test their patience, faith, hope, and love, to develop in them these things.

A visitor may be sent to "receive" from a sick person ministries of consolation, help or warning. If it is plainly marked out that it is your duty to see someone, that you are called to do so, then do not avoid the suffering. It may cost you precious energy but deliver it as you have often done before, as a *"living sacrifice"* (Romans 12:1 AV). Ask God to bless the visit in whatever way He sees best: *"Do not neglect to show hospitality to strangers, for thereby some have entertained angels unawares"* (Hebrews 13:2).

Some people will tell you that you look particularly well, just when you are suffering the most. Others say, "How much better you look than when I saw you last!" when you know and feel that you have been growing worse.

Some say , "You look so much better than I expected to see you; your eyes are so bright, and you look so cheerful, you cannot surely be suffering as much as you say", when you well know how great the effort is to be cheerful. The Enemy offers the thought to you, "Am I then to be punished for the very things which I do because it seems to me a Christian duty to do them?"

No, not punished, but tested. Satan tempted Job, but God permitted it, for his profit, and so it is with you. Do not be downhearted. No two people will give the same opinion of your appearance or state. Some will tell you that you look better, to cheer you, others, from ignorance, because they do not remember how you looked when they saw you last.

They think they have to say something. Others will do it because of their own mood of mind at the time. If all things look bright to them, they imagine you look better, or the reverse. Others think that you are "only nervous" and that they can bring you out of it by cheering you up, that you are deceiving yourself and others, by your delusions and imaginings about your health.

People's words and opinions are often very trying to the sick and cause great searching of heart in them. Yet they really ought not to be listened to much, or to cause the sick any distress.

Looks especially, are no real guides. People often look the best when they are the most ill and the reverse. So much depends on natural appearance or complexion, and on many other causes.

Do not think your friends unloving or unkind, if they never ask how you are, or show any anxiety about you. Some people do this in mistaken kindness. They think that it only brings your illness before you or pains you or annoys you. It is true that some sick people have a great dislike of being asked how they are, for various reasons. Sometimes, it is from a mere feeling of despondency, almost despair. They have only the same or a worse tale to tell and they hate the tale. Sometimes, it is from a dislike of being reminded of their state. Sometimes it is because they fancy that it shows an absence of selfishness not to speak of them. Sometimes, it is that they do not want their illness to be known or talked of and will not therefore put people in possession of any means of doing so. Some draw back from being noticed or have complaints that they wish to conceal.

All these are 'morbid' feelings and the last two often lead to deception. It is best to answer briefly and simply. It is easy to see whether people ask, for the sake of politeness or because they take a real interest in you. Give to the former as brief an answer as is consistent with courtesy. Answer the questions of the latter as they are asked, kindly and freely and, as soon as you can, politely, change the conversation.

Do not get into a habit of talking much of yourself or of your complaints. It is very harmful and produces a habit of self-contemplation, which makes you burdensome to others and the habit will grow. There are times when it is good to talk about yourself with those who well understand us and can analyse our feelings for us, those who can advise us and will rebuke us when we are self-indulgent.

Try to cultivate self-control in all your words, looks, and actions. Do not show the pain you are suffering, more than you can help in your expression, as it is surprising how much habit and discipline may do on this point. Be very careful also how you describe your pain. Never exaggerate it in anyway for this is sure to increase its reality for you. Also, exaggeration is sin.

Conceal your pain from general observers as much as you can, in word, look, and action. Do not count your friends unloving if they tell you off, or even if they seem to you to scold you sharply. Receive their reproofs as the truest token of love and faithfulness, *"Faithful are the wounds of a friend"* (Proverbs 27:6). Would they show their love by *"suffering sin upon you"* (Leviticus 19:17)?

Your first impulse may be to resent it or to think it is very unkind and insensitive, adding to your suffering instead of trying to lessen it. Or you may be tempted to answer fretfully and angrily. If you do, you will probably deprive yourself of the blessing another time.

Sick people are sometimes upset by anyone saying it possible that they can be in a wrong state of mind or are indulging in wrong reactions. Sometimes they think that everyone *ought* to bear with whatever faults they exhibit and that they have enough excuse for them, in their pain or in the trials of illness.

Would you put this plea or excuse before God on the "*great and dreadful day of Judgement?*" (Joel 2:31) How then can you use it now? Is not the present time the season of preparation for that awful hour? Is not your sickness sent to help you in preparation for that? Would you then refuse this good gift of God, by making it an excuse for sin?

No, surely you will seek to be more and more thankful to those friends who imitate the example of the Church and teach that exhortation[48] is the true comfort.

Do not measure the love of your friends by their words, or always by their deeds, but take each person naturally, according to their characters. Expect nothing from them but what is reasonable, which is to be judged of by their habits. Do not expect them to depart from these for you, or to look upon their not doing so as any personal slight.

If you are in the house with many people, some of them may rarely come to see you, unless some special occasion brings them. Others may come daily or more frequently. Do not judge them by these things but by what you know of their character as a whole. Seek to be as little upset by these things as you possibly can be, which will be far beyond what you can imagine, until you try to learn and practice self-discipline.

Do not express disappointment at friends not coming more frequently to see you, except to those people to whom you see that your doing so gives pleasure, and makes them feel that you like their society. At any rate, do not show that it has given you pain. For, if your friends are shy, reserved, or lazy and these have been the causes of their absence, you will only drive them further from you and hinder pleasant conversation when you can have it but it will give an awkwardness and constraint both to yourself and to them.

---

[48]Exhortation means admonishing, urging someone to do what is good.

Sickness: its Trials and Blessings

Be careful not to find fault or to be displeased, if your friends do not tell you everything that happens in the family or all that interests them. Believe that it is their wish to give you pleasure but if they forget to tell you things. it is the same for them as for you. They forget what they intended to say at the right time, when they are with you.

Do not think them unkind if they do not always propose to see you when they visit. You cannot expect always and at all times to be borne in mind. With the kindest and best friend this will not happen, except very rarely. It will spoil all your relationship with your friends and be as much for your trial, as for theirs, if you expect such a thing.

Be very thankful and show yourself pleased whenever any kindness, however trivial, is shown to you, whenever, in any way you are drawn into the range of their pleasures and pursuits. Always accept each thing cheerfully and pleasantly. Nothing is so likely to secure a repetition of the pleasure. If it is not quite agreeable or convenient to you or what you like, try to hide that, and accept the good will of your friend.

When friends come to visit you, this also has its trials. Sometimes you may have made a great effort to see them, and in body and mind be painfully conscious of the effort. You may feel that you have intended it as a kindness towards them or you may have done some act of kindness and it may fall quite flat. Do not be discouraged, as such trials are common to mankind. Sick people cannot expect to be exempt from them.

Or you may begin a conversation, hoping to find it a subject of great interest to your friend, as it is, perhaps, to you. Or it may be some subject which is deeply interesting to you at the time, but it may be received coldly or abstractedly, or dropped at once, as if it had no meaning in it for your friend. These things are a great trial but receive them as such. Do not let them make you morose or discontented or selfishly shut up in yourself, so that you do not want to reach out again, in case you should but suffer rejection and pain.

Do not say, "I have enough trial without this. Surely they might remember that I am ill, cut off from the pleasures of society, from general relationships". No, you have not enough or this would not have been added. It is only life that you are experiencing. You are tried in this way less frequently than others who come into constant contact with many people.

Remember this : "*Love bears all things*" (1 Corinthians 13:7). Remember too, that mere sickness does not exercise us in many necessary points. It is these added trials that test us. They are "*to humble us*" (Deuteronomy 8:2). Besides, you say that you wish to have more participation in life. Do not draw back from a share in these "lesser sharpness of our common grieves". Do not think your friends unreasonable if they expect too much from you. Perhaps they expect, or they seem to you to think, that they shall never see any indication of discontent, irritability or lack of cheerfulness in you.

They think that illness is sent to do you good and they expect to see the good crop springing up in what is really the seed-time. If they are true friends, they may, perhaps, rebuke you, not, as it seems to you, very reasonably and gently. Either you grow angry, or else you say in your heart, "How unreasonable! Surely sickness only stirs up all the evil that is in me and does not subdue it. It is very hard when I am struggling all the day long that I should meet with such unreasonable treatment". It is indeed a very trying but is it quite as unreasonable as it seems to you?

If your friend has not been in your circumstances, can she or he grasp them? She or he is reasoning using the common belief that sick people ought to be gentler and more loving and to demonstrate the fruits of the Spirit more than others do. To a great extent this is true, but, like most statements, it is not the whole truth.

Do not think them unkind, if they urge you to make an effort which you feel to be quite beyond your power. Do not resent it as unkindness, but believe that it was intended for your real good. Perhaps it was made by the fear of your falling into greater depths of illness, or the fear of your becoming a confirmed invalid, or, what is worse, a neurotic patient. Listen to them quietly and patiently. Say gently that you have often made such attempts and always find yourself the worse for them, but that you will gladly try again if they wish it, or you will ask your Physician's advice about it, at the first opportunity. If you are really aware that you are doing the utmost that you have power to do then just be content to be misunderstood and take it patiently. Tell everything to Him who never misunderstands and who reads your heart.

Do not expect friends to tell you every little thing that you would like to hear. Perhaps they have mentioned these things already to other people and may not recall that they have not mentioned them to you, or their minds may are distracted.

They may have had the intention of telling you something, or bringing you some letter or some new book, or something that they think will interest you but it escapes their memory just at the time they leave home to come to you.

Believe in the love of your friends and rest in that. It will be the greatest help to you. *"Judge not, that you be not judged"* (Matthew 7:1).

2.19 Letters[49] and Communications

Sometimes letters and any kind of communication are a source of emotional discontent or disturbance to the sick.

---

[49]We have taken the liberty to render 'letters' together with 'communications' so that readers can mentally transfer the phrase "letters" to whatever means they use to communicate with others.

Sickness: its Trials and Blessings

We have spoken of the pleasure of receiving communications and how welcome they are. Sometimes, however, if a friend does not write as much as the sick person would like of his illness, or does not seem to enter into it or seems to misunderstand the illness completely and thinks the sick person can do 'such and such' when he or she is longing to do so, but cannot, or thinks that the sick person ought to try to make this and many other exertion or perhaps judges them harshly, then such communications can become a source of irritation. It is fortunate if a cooling of the relationship is not an outcome.

All these things are sent to 'try' us. They are intended to. Nevertheless, we should bear in mind that we ought not to be angry or even annoyed and that our friend meant nothing but kindness. However, being at a distance and unable to see us, he or she could not possibly know our actual circumstances. They wrote, either judging from our own statements, from the statements of others, or from having formed an imaginary picture of what state such and such symptoms would probably produce.

Just as you do not like to be harshly judged, do not judge your friend harshly. Be very careful not to answer in an irritated tone, or to let an unkind word escape you. If you feel upset, do not write at once. Wait until the first feeling of irritation and upset and its after-thoughts have subsided.

Ask the God of Love to make you more Himself and to make this a time for denying yourself and to enable you to hide from your friend that you have done so. You can naturally and quietly tell them your state; but do not try to make it appear worse or different from what it really is, for that would be but another way of expressing your annoyance.

Sick people often expect their friends to communicate with them as frequently and as fully as if they can write answering each letter. This is unreasonable. It is not likely that people who are healthy can fully enter into the feelings of sick persons about communication. They feel so cut off from life that they often have a craving for contact, if not for communications, but a great disinclination to, or inability to answer them.

A communication steals into the room so silently and quietly that it does not fatigue one as visitors sometimes do. It gives great pleasure to find that friends remember us and do not stop writing to us, even when we cannot acknowledge the cheer their communications have been to us.

People often say, "I do not write to you, because I know how weak you are and that it only burdens you". This is a great mistake. Sick people need communication more, in order to keep up their connection with others and they value it far more than healthy people do. If people are afraid to tire the sick, they should say that they do not expect answers and will write again, in spite of not receiving any reply. Never reproach sick people for not replying, or think it is proof of lack of affection. Similarly, let the sick remember how often their friends abstain from writing to them from truly kind motives and so never indulge unloving thoughts of them.

Unless they have been ill for a long time, few people can fully understand the enjoyment of receiving a handwritten lette, and even those often uncared for messages of love and remembrance.

2.20 Visits of the Clergy and Christian Ministers

Another source of discontent often arises from the visits of the clergy and Christian ministers. You may be living in a large parish where it is not possible for your pastor to visit you often. He has so large a fold and so many sheep to look after.

Remember that you are not the only one and that his time is greatly occupied. Be thankful then, whenever he visits you and be thankful also when he does not, if you know that it is because he is visiting others who have fewer means of Christian instruction and have had only a few opportunities of obtaining it.

Or, you may be living in a parish where the people are rarely visited. If so, your case is not peculiar. You have no cause to complain, as if you were worse off than others. Pray for yourself and those shut in, that the case may become otherwise, if it so pleases God.

Or a Minister visits you and the conversation may be entirely desultory, about people or on general subjects. Or, the Minister may be very shy and reserved and feel deeply that he does not know how to address you. He may have an earnest desire to but feeling this difficulty may make his manner cold or formal. You find that you can say nothing. You had questions you wanted to ask, advice to get from him but you are restrained. You ask nothing. He leaves you and you say in your heart, with bitter disappointment, that your *"teachers are removed into a corner"* (Isaiah 30:20).

Or, he may know nothing, personally, of illness and may not have much studied the wants of the sick, which may be learned by an earnest study of the "Service for the Visitation of the Sick." He thinks, perhaps, that all the needs of sick people are alike, all their trials all coming under the same class, that what he says to one will equally apply to every case.

Perhaps he is as much surprised that his words do not seem to suit you, as you are that he says nothing which comes 'home to your heart'. He may have a method in his visits which you would interrupt if you asked any question. You see that it is not agreeable to him: it breaks the train of his thought, which he cannot easily resume. He has adopted this course with the sick, considerately, believing it to be the plan most likely to edify them.

Even when, before he leaves, he proposes to read a chapter from Holy Scripture and then to pray with you, he did not

Sickness: its Trials and Blessings

perceive your weakness. He did not notice that you could not now listen or follow as once you could and that you needed the Scripture read to you and that the Prayer should be adapted to your physical condition, if you are to take part in it. Perhaps you are not able to have more than two or three prayers or Collects repeated, the words of which you are so familiar with, as to require only the one effort of joining in the prayer, without considering what words were said and whether you could join in. You expected so much from this visit and yet you are disappointed and you feel more alone and lacking in help than before.

Or, the pastor may think something that you say is erroneous and spend his visit in combating the error, rather than in leading you into truth. Or, he may expect you to respond to certain words and phrases but you are afraid to express yourself like this. The words do not exactly convey your meaning. You give a wrong impression of yourself ; you say that you cannot use such words. He is dissatisfied. Perhaps he tells you that *"The root of the matter is found in you"* (Job 19:28) or that you "have departed from first principles." You are discouraged. Perhaps you really meant the same thing that he did, but you felt that you have often used such words without any meaning and that sickness especially had revealed this sin to you and now you cannot truly express yourself precisely, although you feel you meant the same thing. You were just afraid of appearing better than you feel yourself to be.

Or, it may be that you were confused or frightened, because you had not been accustomed to be asked so many questions about your own inmost thoughts. You may have had many things on your mind to speak about, or questions to ask, but you felt that you would not be understood. Or, you may have an entirely formal visit and you are made to feel that it is so completely a matter of 'business' that you find it hard to take any part in it.

Sickness: its Trials and Blessings

If you are actually living in the house of a Minister of Religion, you will perhaps see many pastors but will not, often, probably, be much better off for pastoral visits. Generally, they will tell you that they do not come to "visit" you, but merely come as a friend; that they know how well you are already provided for in your own house and much better visited than you can be by others. It is a natural supposition. But when it is remembered that if you are one of the family of a Pastor and he has much to do, he will rarely have time to bestow on you.

Your father or husband, if he is a Minister, thinks that he can see you at any time but when you see him, there are often so many personal and domestic subjects to be spoken of that all the very little time is absorbed in them. You know that he is ever ready at hand and in any emergency you would ask his help, but you, of anyone, perhaps best knows how over tasked his strength is. It would be a mere pain to you to add any weight to his burden. Moreover, it rarely happens that members of a family can so throw aside other relationships as to easily merge all in the Shepherd and the sheep. They may offer delightful spiritual conversations, but not exactly pastoral care. Therefore do not expect what, in fact, cannot be.

What you want is to be encouraged by your Minister to lay your troubles and difficulties before him and to receive his counsel and help. You want to feel that you shall be understood and that you may have perfect confidence in him, without any fear that your words will ever be heard by anyone else. You want to meet with ready sympathy, not a dry, cold, abstracted hearing, or by a misunderstanding of your words. You want to feel that whatever you say which is wrong, he will point out to you, not supposing some error in you which does not exist. You do not want him to talk to you of "the errors of the present day" and warn you against them, but to point out your own errors. You want to have sin pointed out to you, to have plain, honest truth spoken, to be exhorted, more than comforted. You do not want to be merely told of the blessings of sickness and that *"The Lord disciplines the one he loves, and chastises every son whom he receives"* (Hebrews 12:6) but to learn that illness is a chastisement.

You want to be directed how practically to "believe in the Holy Catholic Church and the Communion of Saints[50]" and to be shown how truly you are still a member of the Church and not cut off, though a 'sick member'. You want to know how you are "still preserved in the unity of the Church"[51]. You want to be instructed in the best way of joining all the members of the Church and how to be sure that services of the church are for the sick, as well as for those who can go to church. You feel that there are *"green pastures and still waters"* (Psalms 23:2) and you want to be led *"by them"*. You want to be told what your 'part' and 'duty' is and how to *"fulfil your course"* (Acts 3:25) so that the *"whole body, joined and held together by every joint"* (Ephesians 4:16) do that which is appointed for it to do.

It is a great help in profiting from the visits of pastors to remember that they are *"God's ministers"* (Romans 13:6), His servants. They come to us in another character from ordinary men. They are called by God, as Aaron was (Hebrews 5:4). Like Moses, they may be *"slow of speech and of slow tongue"* (Exodus 4:10). They are *"men of like passions"* (Acts 14:15) yet they have a special work and calling which fits them to be teachers. The more willing we are to learn from

---

[50] The Creed

[51] This sentence comes from the Church of England's Confession of Sin and the form of absolution implies the restoration after excommunication of a sick member of the church, meaning a member who has been disciplined having transgressed some church rule, so it restores the member into communion. For 'sick member', Priscilla Maurice may have understood that the person cut off means someone literally sick, instead as it is meant, someone who is 'morally sick' and so excluded from the Church, by its discipline.

them and to *"Remember your leaders, those who spoke to you the word of God. Consider the outcome of their way of life, and imitate their faith"* (Hebrews 13:7) the more we shall find that they do bring us a message. To this message *"you will do well to pay attention as to a lamp shining in a dark place"* (2 Peter 1:19).

We can learn much from Ministers whose words are not pleasing to our taste. We ignore many excellent words because they do not seem to suit us at the time. We are provoked by them because they may not suit us. But the day may come when the words they spoke will return to us and *"leave a blessing behind"* (Joel 2:14).

2.21 Medical Advice and Medical Visits

There is another trial which often gives rise to feelings of discontent in the minds of the chronically sick. It shows itself in two opposite ways.

Sometimes those who are sick think that because their friends let them carry on without wishing they should seek additional medical advice or a change of doctor, they do not care for their recovery or do not wish them to try alternatives. This idea preys upon their minds and gives them a feeling of deep dissatisfaction. Were the sick to speak the truth, or rather, if they knew their own hearts, they would see how much they themselves are wanting to try some new treatment or to have a new doctor.

Visitors often propose this course of action and urge them to try someone in whom they can have special confidence. Perhaps this stirs up the desire in their minds and even produces a feeling of dissatisfaction with their present treatment? The sick person ponders it in his or her heart and wonders why his or her supporters are so indifferent to the idea.

It is the love and kindness of friends, generally speaking, that makes them think like this. They see that little or nothing can be done and they kindly forbear to frustrate their sick friend by asking them to try fresh treatments which may only make them worse and in the end, cause disappointment.

They think it kinder to leave them to the soothing remedies which are generally resorted to when all others are ineffectual, than to put them to the pain of undergoing many of the same remedies that have been tried already, without success.

So if you wish to see some new doctor, propose it yourself. At least tell a friend that you think you should like to have such advice and if they see no objection. But always remember when you are doing so, how great a risk you are running.

The advice you seek may not suit you at all and it may merely add to your suffering[52]. You cannot expect that a stranger should take the interest in you that someone would who has long watched your case and known you. His or her 'manner' may be trying to you and his opinion of your case cause you fresh distress.

Weigh all these things carefully. Some sick people are constantly wishing for a change of medical advisers. What do they gain by it? A succession of disappointments and trials? Medicines given and rejected as failures, hope after hope arising, and as often failing.

In the early stage of an illness, it is very desirable to have more than one medical opinion; but when all options have been tried, it is a far more peaceful to stick to one doctor,

---

[52]We have seen patients who have spent previous financial resources on numerous kinds of healers and doctors and yet get no better. They do this rather than ask God alone to guide them which doctor to consult (which is our strong advice). We are surprised that Priscilla Maurice does not advise praying for the right doctor, herself.

Sickness: its Trials and Blessings

whoever suits you best and not to seek for, or hanker for any more opinions. There are stages in a disease in which it may be well, if your usual doctor approves it, to have a fresh opinion but the less frequently the better. Some sick people have a foolish desire for any new medical opinion[53].

If friends wish and propose it, it is your duty to fall in with their wishes and give them the satisfaction of having tried all reasonable means. If they do not care about urging this, then you may be content and thankful. But do not be displeased if they express their wish that you should see some fresh person. Take it as a proof of kindness. Do not be discontented, or think that they are upsetting you needlessly.

Sometime, the sick are discontented with their doctor because he offers no treatment that works for them. But surely this is not a just cause for discontent? We can be assured that every honest medically trained person will desire to cure their patient and if he or she cannot, at least to offer all the relief in his or her power.

Sometimes, sick people think that doctors do not understand their particular case. Perhaps they do not, because they are working in the dark. But is this just cause for discontent? Could not He who opened the eyes of the blind, open their eyes to see your case clearly and give them understanding to treat it?

Ask advice from some friends on whom you can rely. Ask if your case seems to them as it does to you, and if their opinion agrees with yours. If they advise that you should seek another medical opinion, then do it. But if this cannot be done, then take it as His will that you are not to be relieved,

---

[53]Some believers do, indeed, drain their bank accounts by taking the latest fashionable and costly 'healing', course or alternative treatment particularly if they discovered the treatment on the internet. Nor do they seem to care when these treatments are useless. All that seems to matter is taking the initiative by consulting the internet and not the will of God through faith and prayer.

Sickness: its Trials and Blessings

and as His will that you must still suffer. This will soften the situation for you and enable you to receive the trial meekly.

Sometimes we feel that doctors misunderstand our characters. They urge some people, whose whole mind and spirit is active, to even greater effort and to whom stillness is a greater suffering and trial than any of their remedies. But by doing so, they increase the restlessness and discontent in their patients.

Or, sometimes doctors let those who need to be roused and stirred up, remain idle. The reason is that they know little of their patients and they are rarely acquainted with them before their illness. Therefore they cannot know their natural characters. They only hear our tales of illness, which we feel it necessary to tell them fully, and they think that these are our thoughts at all times, the natural 'food' of our minds. Hence they judge that we need to be brought out of what seems to them 'morbid'. Therefore they urge us, in kindness, but indiscriminately. Many doctors have cultivated a knowledge of disease more than a knowledge of human nature. They look at the face as the index of the disease, rather than at the mind, within.

Another of the great trials which doctors often cause their patients is treating them (not medically, perhaps, but morally) as a having a mere 'nervous' illness. Do they not know, we sometimes ask, that they can say nothing more hopeless and discouraging to a sick person? If they mean, "It is nothing, do not think of it, try to forget it," surely these words will not produce the effect they intend?

Instead of this, they could say, "These are morbid feelings and you must struggle against them. They can be overcome. It will cost you a great and continued struggle, but you will be rewarded for doing so". Then there would be hope and strength in such language and the work given you to do would be very useful. The sick person would value the friend who speaks such truth to him.

On the other hand, the effect of saying, "It is only a nervous illness" is to prevent the sufferer from uttering their real thoughts, or any similar ones in order to prevent them being so wrongly construed. They make their doctor feel that he does not understand him and they shake his confidence in his opinions, even when there is no ground for it. Yet the doctor should remember that he merely used a common term and did not intend to cause so much pain.

If, on the other hand, he means by "merely nerves," or "neurotic pain", an affection of the nerves, then his words are sad and hopeless. No pains are so peculiarly trying, so inexplicable, so incurable. But if this is the meaning of his words, then surely it is better to be told? It is better to know the whole, sad truth, to be able to face it all and to see what it involves and to seek how to meet it in the strength of the Lord.

Do not trouble your doctor with questions about his opinion of your state, the nature of the disease or its prognosis. You will gain nothing by doing so. He will perhaps argue from such questions that you spend a great deal of your time thinking about it. Except when any particular changes occur in the disease, he knows nothing new and he can tell you nothing except what he has already told you. Instead, you may tempt him to give you some unwelcome opinion as to its duration, or your degree of nervousness.

Better to go on patiently, from week to week, asking no questions and just living in the day and for the day, feeling that after all, your life is not in your doctor's hands, but in God's who *"wounds, but he binds up; he shatters, but his hands heal"* (Job 5:18).

Always answer all questions asked by doctors clearly, distinctly, truly and without any reservations. But the less you volunteer about your bodily feelings the better, unless there are any necessary things to be mentioned which these ques-

Sickness: its Trials and Blessings

tions have not elicited. In this case, describe them in as few words as possible.

Do not conceal any symptoms from doctors. It is a mistake even if there is modesty in doing so. It may be a great trial to you to speak of some embarrassing things and to submit to some treatments, but take it as a trial. It is part of your discipline and a necessary and humbling one. Do not make objections to trying treatments. It is your duty to try whatever is suggested. Do not say that you cannot take this or that medicine. Try it again. Under your present circumstances the effect may be quite different to what the effect was before. You owe it to your doctor to try anything which he thinks may be useful to you.

The manner in which some doctors talk to the friends of the sick, causes much trial to sick people. They may speak of them as 'psychological ill', saying that they must be treated as such, be urged to make an effort and told that they have no organic disease. This often causes others not only to think too lightly of the illness, but inflict great suffering on the sick person by acting in accordance with the medical opinion, irrespective of their own instinctive knowledge of the characters of their friends.

Another trial which a long illness frequently brings is that doctors grow weary of the case. At first they are deeply interested in it, but it will not yield to their remedies. Then they grow impatient with it, call it 'psychological' and then perhaps even ridicule the very ailments. They may make their visits less and less frequently, until, on one side or the other, the attendance ends. This is a sore trial, for the suffering neither ends nor diminishes, but goes on its weary way, the strength, nerves and heart, meanwhile, giving way.

Such trials should teach us to value deeply the long, unwearied, patient, faithful kindness of some medical friend, who has continued, in spite of all discouragements, to visit us still, not in the expectation of cure, but just in the hope of alleviating, soothing and comforting. Such doctors will, indeed: *"by no means lose his reward"* (Matthew 10:42). They shall be *"repaid at the resurrection of the just"* (Luke 14:14). They shall surely find, even now, that *"Blessed is the one who considers the poor! In the day of trouble the Lord delivers him"* (Psalms 41:1).

People are apt to extol those who cure them. But how much more praise and gratitude do those doctors deserve who do not have this reward of their skill? Those who are not blessed with these good gifts from God may, at least, take comfort that the Great Physician God, *"Does not faint or grow weary; His understanding is unsearchable"* (Isaiah 40:28).

Though no other hand may pour oil or wine into your wounds[54], God Himself will do it and He who has sent the pain, and all its innumerable trials, will stand by at all times, to soothe, and cheer, strengthen and bless you. "Drink then with the patience of the Saints and the God of Love will bless the physic"[55].

2.22 Nurses and Carers

Another class of the trials which weakness brings comes from nurses and carers. The innumerable ideas which haunt a sick person on this subject cannot be easily described.

---

[54] This is a Bible expression coming from one of Jesus parables: *"And went to him, and bound up his wounds, pouring in oil and wine, and set him on his own beast, and brought him to an inn, and took care of him"* (Luke 10:34). Oil and wine were also considered medicine, in antiquity.

[55] A quotation from a letter by Samuel Rutherford to Viscountess of Kenmore who was suffering from spiritual depression. Samuel Rutherford's letters are full of counsel to the afflicted. Tender compassion and strong counsel are distinguishing features throughout his Letters. Samuel Rutherford (1600? – 1661) was a Scottish Presbyterian theologian and author. He was one of the Scottish Commissioners to the Westminster Assembly.

Sickness: its Trials and Blessings

Sometimes you may take a most violent dislike to some carer. This dislike may be quite without reason, but it seems impossible to overcome. The sick person feels that it is, perhaps, very sinful, and earnestly fights against it but in vain. The more he or she strives, the stronger it grows.

Each time this person enters the room, the patient grows restless and distressed and, if he or she comes near the bed or sofa, it is only by the mercy of God that some words of annoyance or displeasure do not burst out. At any rate, it may cause really distressing feelings, quicken the pulse, make the heart beat quickly or even seem to stop. There may be a sensation of not being able to breathe when this person is nearby, as if he or she took up all the air you ought to have. The person seems to oppress you, to be a weight on your heart or our spirits. You feel bullied and long for the carer to leave.

Or what is far more distressing, it may be some dear friend, towards whom you feel such feelings and you cannot account for it at all. You only know that you feel that they are not what you want, now. They seem to provoke you, by their awkwardness. They cannot do anything for you, except, as it seems to you, very clumsily. They seldom give you the thing that you want or ask for, or in the way you long for it. They ask what you want, where to find it and how they should give it until you, feeling that they ought to know all this and not trouble you, get anxious and upset. You think how little they do for you and say that you had rather not have what you want than to be forced to give so many directions. If such a person should chance to sit up at night with you, you feel given over to discomfort for the whole night. They cannot do a single thing which is pleasing. You do not try to seem pleased and they lose heart.

On the other hand, perhaps there is some friend or carer whom you particularly like. No one else can put your pillows comfortably. No one else can give you medicines, even

Sickness: its Trials and Blessings

the smallest thing that you need. If anyone else brings you your food, you do not like it and feel neglected. You will not be pleased and satisfied, however kindly and well the thing may be done by someone else.

In this situation there are temptations and just as in the former case, there is the danger of over tasking the strength of your carer, of taxing his or her power and laying heavy burdens on others. The kinder he or she is, the more willingness to do what you wish, the greater your danger.

Be very careful that you are not over-demanding towards your helpers. Consider them always as you would like to be considered. Never wear them out, just because you do not like anyone else to wait on you, because this is very selfish. Again, there is the danger that other people will be grieved at your partiality for someone because you will not let them do anything for you, or show their desire to help you.

It is a great duty in illness to avoid putting others to pain in this way. Besides which, instead of them being drawn closer in love and sympathy with you by your illness, you push them further away.

When you feel this temptation, say, to dislike your carer, perhaps it may be of some help to you to:

1. avoid speaking speak of it to anyone.

2. redouble your efforts to show kindness to that person, in thought, word, and manner, and especially, to pray for them.

3. avoid reasoning about it but put the thought away untouched, whenever it offers itself to your mind.

4. lay it before God and tell Him how very much it distresses you, that you cannot overcome it, but that you hate yourself for it. Go on doing so continually. Say "*Father, if it be possible, let this cup pass from me*". But if not, then ask Him to teach you to say,

"Your will be done". Then take it as His will and this will change the nature of the trial. Bear it submissively until He sees fit to remove it from you.

There may be some cases in which a nurse sent by an agency may really be unsuitable. Therefore it is better to speak to some friend about it and, if it seems to them the same way, it is best to make a change of carer, as soon as possible. We may receive the most helpful discipline from the various characters of our attendants, if we decide to. Otherwise they will only fret us and stir up the evil which is inside us.

We need not seek out those people who will test us. On the contrary, it is far better for them and for us, that we should choose those who seem likely to suit us. But in every character we shall find something not quite according to our liking so let us take this as wholesome discipline and use it as such.

Are you very impatient and impetuous, by nature? Your helper may be valuable to you and yet she may be a continual chastisement to you, by reason of her slowness. It is very discouraging to her and bad for you, that you should be constantly telling her off for it or trying to hurry her. Take it as a means of correcting the evil that is in you and it will prove to be the case. Few things can so constantly remind you of your besetting sin, and warn you to correct it.

Most of all watch your tone and manner. Your greatest temptation to speak evil comes out in how you treat your helpers and nurses. We are apt to give sad license to ourselves with those whose job it is to tend us, not merely forgetting how much we must test their patience and hurt them, but also what an example we are setting to them, and how we are weakening, if not destroying, the influence that we might have, and ought to have, over them.

What if they are slow, unintelligent, unreliable or misunderstand us, seem indifferent, are forgetful, selfish, or unwilling to be put out of their way? Let us ask ourselves if we are never like that too?

Have we never found any of the faults in ourselves that we complain of, in them? Have we tried hard, by example, kindness, gentle rebuke, patience and forbearance, to overcome their faults in them? Do we never make them angry and therefore call out the evil in them?

Have we asked God to teach us how to help them, to bear with them and to lead them in a better way? Do we ask this, day by day and whenever we come in contact with them? Many people will speak sharply or impatiently to a helper or nurse who would not do so to a friend. Perhaps there is no check more wholesome than watching one's words and ways for they are with us when no one else is and at the times we are least on our guard, when only His eye sees and His ear hears. He will call us to account for these things, as well as all *"things done in the body"* (2 Corinthians 5:10 AV).

You will also be careful not to burden your carer unnecessarily, not to call for attention unreasonably frequently, or when you can do without the thing you wanted. Perhaps it is something which can wait until she next comes. You will be careful never to disturb her rest at night unnecessarily, to consider her own health and comfort; to allow her proper exercise in the open air, which those who attend closely on the sick especially need. If she has been up in the night, you will take care that she has rest in the day. You will always consider her meal time and not let it be needlessly interrupted. You will always try to show to her that you are satisfied and grateful to her. Those who wait on the sick need a great deal of patience. If she does not please you, it is best occasionally to speak only very kindly to her. Avoid constantly making little complaints and finding fault with everything; for that is so discouraging, that you cannot expect her to respond well.

You will decide also to resist all desires, which though, perhaps not wrong in themselves, may be very inconvenient or expensive to your friends but which they may not like to deny you. Remember, *"If anyone would come after me, let him deny himself and take up his cross and follow me"* (Matthew 16:24). These are your Master's words to you.

2.23 Being a Burden

Do not distress yourself by thinking "I am just a burden". How often sick people say this. How often they think this and the thought is, indeed, a distressing one. It is a blessing if the thought develops no further and does not degenerate into thinking that our friends think the same thoughts that we have in our own minds. In other words that they think us troublesome and are growing weary of us.

These thoughts sometimes occupy the thoughts of every sick person. It is right that you should constantly try to bear in mind how great the trial is for those around you. The more tenderly they love you, the greater it must be. Besides, the sorrow that your sickness causes your friends, there is also a peculiar sense of depression which pervades a household during sickness, especially if it is a short and dangerous one.

Generally speaking, the habits of a family are upset by illness, and to some extent changed. One is missed from one's accustomed place in the circle and from family meetings. When any of the family have been out, still to find sickness meeting them on their return, gives sadness. They can never take refreshment away from illness, for it is 'pressing' on them at home. But do not let the thought of this depress you. Instead ask that it may make you more loving, gentle, and considerate, and thankful to all those around you. Let it remain alive during the rest of your life, as a grateful remembrance.

Sickness: its Trials and Blessings

There are many ways in which you can avoid giving trouble, if you are really determined to do so and you are not merely indulging in morbid thoughts and words. You can be constantly avoiding giving trouble without any appearance of doing so. You will, of course, try as much as possible, to let your hours and habits harmonise with those around. You will take your meals at the same time, when it is possible, and make your free and leisure times those which will best suit other people. As little as possible shut out the family from your room. Do not make it a 'favour' to receive them. Do not show that you feel they are 'in the way'. They come to you in kindness, so receive them kindly and cheerfully.

Perhaps it may help you when the fear of giving trouble distresses you, to clearly to run over these things in your mind:

- Is it really a dislike of giving trouble, free of other feelings? Is there no pride in not wanting to give trouble? Is there no feeling of being a taker, and not a giver? Is there no dislike of dependence and a self-centred striving for independence in your feeling?

- The spiritual 'message' issuing from your illness is for your friends and relatives as well as for yourself. You must not fear that you should seem a kind of messenger of evil tidings. Even if they look upon it as a kind of intrusion on their comfort, putting into disarray their agendas and destroying their enjoyment, then they need the message the more, and you must be content to be the bearer of it.

- You did not bring yourself into these circumstances. Instead, it was the will of God. He is too wise to order His discipline, that it shall bless one person and injure another of His children. Be assured that what is sent to bless you and to teach you, is sent to bless and to teach all your relatives and friends too. Do not say that you are 'in the way', that you are causing so many burdens and give so much trouble, while being unable to move a

Sickness: its Trials and Blessings

hand or foot to help. You are God's messenger. Leave it to Him to apply the message to the hearts of everyone. But do not ruin it, by trying to persuade yourself or others that it is your message and that you bring it very unwillingly. The greeting which the Church appoints that pastors visiting the sick should give is "Peace be to this house and to all that dwell in it". The Son of Peace is in it. Jesus has sent a messenger to you. Do not be forgetful to entertain this stranger, for hereby some have *"welcomed angels as guests, without even knowing it"* (Hebrews 13:2 CEV).

- The lot that God appoints is good. He has placed you where you are. He has appointed all your circumstances even down to the minutest detail. It is exactly adapted to your character. Nothing else would do what has to be done so well, or teach you so much. Answer every suggestion of Satan, who wants to tempt you to believe that these are not the best circumstances and that others would have suited your character better with, *"Satan, get away from me!"* (Matthew 16:23 CEV). "God has placed me here. It is the will of God." When anyone suggests to you that they wish your circumstances were different, say, *"It is the will of God, the only wise God"* (1 Timothy 1:17) *"our Father"* (Matthew 6:9). When your own heart tempts you, in however small a prompting to persuade you to wish otherwise, say, "It is the will of God" the "God of Love".

2.24 The Temptation to think that no one can sympathize

You must always think of sickness as a hidden state, fully known only to its wayfarers. So take care how you use the words, "No one can sympathise with me and no one understands me". Not only do these words have a chilling effect upon those listening, they diminish their sympathy, however

Sickness: its Trials and Blessings

much they had wished to sympathize. They will also eventually bring upon you the sad reality of having no one who does sympathize with you. It will also have a most damaging effect upon you, as it produces isolation and loneliness of heart.

Few people stop at "No one can can sympathize". Next comes, "No one *will* sympathize". In other words, "I will not let them sympathize, so I will shut myself away". Few say this, in words. But internally, they lay the blame on other people and think they are very badly treated. But if they reject sympathy and always say when it is offered, "You do not understand me and you cannot enter into my trial", gradually, the attempt to offer sympathy will be naturally withdrawn. These patients have brought this bitter trial wholly upon themselves by their own free choice.

So if you see in your friends the wish to sympathize, accept it gratefully, even if you feel that it reaches only a short way into the reality of your need and never plumbs the depth of your trial. Be assured that gradually, if you cherish their sympathy, it will increase and adapt itself, by use, more to your needs. At first, it may be very awkward. The person offering it may feel this as painful about it as you can do. Therefore feel for them! Give them your help and before long you will have theirs. Do not say "In many things you can sympathize, but not in this particular trial". This may be true. Most things must be experienced in order to be fully understood. But do not speak the words out loud as they are so discouraging. Instead tell it all to Him who never fails in understanding, in sympathy or in love.

Kindness is always precious, so do not 'throw it back' on those who offer it. Accept each little token cheerfully and thankfully. Sometimes someone may bring you may be something which you did not wish for just then. Accept the kindness and keep it to yourself. Do not give your friend disappointment, even if it is costly to you. Having shown yourself to be really grateful, you can courteously ask not to have the same thing brought to you again, if you can find some good reason for not doing so.

Do not assume that things are your 'right'. Courteously and thankfully receive each kindness *as a kindness*. Receive each gift, like a book, flowers, or whatever, cheerfully and gratefully. Remember always that all the kindnesses and the love of friends are gifts from the God of Love.

2.25 Irritability

It is a great help and blessing to a sick person to be told when they are manifesting the irritability which is constantly causing them bitter inner conflict and with which either they are maintaining, or they ought to be, one unbroken, arduous resistance. Sometimes, without any apparent cause, this irritability will suddenly seem to seize one's whole body and every nerve will be strained with the wretched feeling.

Only God knows how long this irritability has been suppressed or how often it has risen up before and has been suppressed. The temptation to anger has been repressed, perhaps, for hours. No trace of irritability has been seen by others. Then some minor mishap occurs. Perhaps this is so minor that you hardly feel it necessary to guard against it. It may be that a door was shut violently, or not shut at all, or held in the hand for some minutes whilst another person outside is being spoken to and you have the double annoyance of expectation and of hearing a whispering sound in which you cannot take part. Or it may be a sudden noisy interruption, something carelessly dropped. Or it may be that someone has forgotten to do something which you particularly wanted them to do. Or, someone suddenly touches you, or your bed, shaking the bed continually whilst sitting by or on it. Or someone comes into the room, unexpectedly, and in a fluster.

These things are too small to name, but not too small to feel. They may have caused a sudden explosion of irritability. The truth is that you may have been exerting yourself beyond your strength. The last ounce of strength has been spent just as this new demand comes upon you. It was too much for your strength which failed.

Be assured that your frustration may be a mere physical expression of nervous suffering and not counted 'sin' by Him who is "very pitiful".

But your friends can rarely distinguish the context in which you lose your temper. How can they? Can you always, in your own case, distinguish between these things in others? No, you cannot. Therefore do not think friends are being unreasonable or unkind if they criticise or chide you for losing your temper. It is a proof of true love for you.

The effort to repress irritability sometimes gives a pained expression to the voice and expression which is easily misunderstood and therefore should be brought under control, as much as possible. People who are ill and who are seeking to *"take every thought captive to obey Christ"* (2 Corinthians 10:5) will seldom utter an irritable word. Perhaps they scarcely think an irritable thought without being instantly aware of it. But then, what a conflict follows when irritability arises! They ask: what is this sin remaining in me still? Is sinfulness not yet subdued in me? Must I suffer from it, forever? How long shall I go on to dishonour my Lord and Master and to be so unlike Him who *"committed no sin, neither was deceit found in his mouth."* (1 Peter 2:22). Have all my struggles been a lie? Have all my prayers been in vain and unheard?

Be assured that they have not been in vain. They have all been heard and they are all answered hour by hour. God *"puts your tears into His bottle. They are in His Book"* (Psalms 56:8 AV). He know you through and through. It is He who supports you each moment that you are upheld *"to keep you from falling"* (Jude 24 AV).

It is by God's grace that you are kept from sinning more often and if you cling to God, you will find what the Bible says is true: *"My soul clings to you; your right hand upholds me"* (Psalms 63:8) and you will less frequently slide. God will *"Set a guard over your mouth and keep watch over the door of your lips"* (Psalms 141:3) so that you will no sin against Him. But have you not also prayed to Him to *"humble you, testing you to know what was in your heart, whether you would keep his commandments or not"* (Deuteronomy 8:2). Is not this the fulfilment of your prayers? Perhaps you still need to be shown some of the evils in your own heart? Do not then be downhearted when you do see them but ask Him, whenever He leads you into the *"room of pictures"* (Ezekiel 8:12) always to go there with you Himself, in case you should be overwhelmed by the vision.

Make sure you look upon your irritable words as spoken primarily before God: *"Against you, you only, have I sinned and done what is evil in your sight, so that you may be justified in your words and blameless in your judgement"* (Psalms 51:4). If you do not think this, the vexed feeling of having done a wrong thing before a fellow creature, will only minister to self- assertion and pride.

Do not be too downhearted and think that all your efforts have been in vain. Do not be fearful, and anxious about the future: *"Humble yourselves, therefore, under the mighty hand of God so that at the proper time He may exalt you, casting all your anxieties on him, because he cares for you"* (1 Peter 5:6-7).

God knows the intensity of the suffering which irritability causes, especially when it is produced by the state of wrought nerves or by great fatigue. A tone of voice which sounds almost fretful is part, some think, of some states of illness. Certainly sick people very often indulge in a fretful tone of voice, until it becomes habitual. Certainly this tone can be resisted to a great extent and can be almost, if not quite, overcome.

It is most important for the health, both of mind and body, not to yield to this fretful tone at all, but to cultivate instead, a cheerful, calm, thankful voice. At the same time, it must be admitted, that there are states of suffering which do affect the voice, and even, in some cases, give it a sharpness, which is physical, and therefore unavoidable. What we mean here is the habitual tone and sick people can indulge in a tone which they imagine belongs to illness.

As a general rule, if you find that your voice has an unnatural tone, try to subdue it and then you will soon discover what is and what is not under your control. Remember that discontent quickly betrays itself in the tone of voice, facial expression and manner.

Sick people should never look upon themselves as having the privilege to do what is wrong whether in word or deed. Their state gives them no exemption from the continual inner conflict of suppressing sin. Instead, they are set in the midst of sin while being put where they can discern more clearly what is sin. This is because they are in a position in which, if they view their condition properly, all superficiality, gloss and distraction is removed both from them and from all the objects upon which they focus.

2.26 Impatience

Perhaps impatience becomes a problem. It may be that you become impatient with being contradicted and dislike putting up with any opposition to your will. You may wish for something, perhaps, which may be very unreasonable, or inconvenient, or even impossible. Do you want your friends to treat you like a spoiled child and, at the risk of further spoiling you, grant your every desire?

Does it not show in them more true kindness gently to oppose or even to deny you what you have asked? Will you not be grateful to them afterwards, for having been the means of revealing to you your waywardness?

Or, you may be impatient because someone differed in opinion from you, as if there were no possibility of your being mistaken, or of there being two or more points of view, from which the same thing may be viewed.

Sick people who live mostly alone are in great danger of falling into this trap. They frequently live in a world of their own making. They have become so used to their own opinions, their own unchallenged world views and to the way they see things. They can forget that there can be other opinions of the same thing and are perhaps perplexed and threatened by them. This kind of isolation is very damaging to them and, in fact, they should be thankful to hear differences of opinion.

Or, you may have given expression to some impatient word or phrase, which at the moment, may scarcely strike you as it may strike a bystander. For example you say "You take such a long time!" or "I wish you would hurry up" or "Do bring that quickly". They are dangerous phrases to use. Often they mean little or nothing but it is the tone of voice which generally betrays what they really mean. Be thankful to anyone who tells you that this is a bad habit and that you must minister to the impatience of your own heart. *"Keep your heart with all vigilance, for from it flow the springs of life."* (Proverbs 4:23). A habit of repressing such words is the greatest possible help to overcoming the evil.

2.27 Considering Symptoms

Another temptation in illness and indeed in all illness, is constantly to be thinking about and talking about your symptoms, wondering what will be the outcome of each one, asking whether this or that sign is dangerous or what is indicates.

Or, if, in fact, you do not want to get better, the temptation is to consider whether this is the symptom of a fatal illness. How long will it last? Does it prove you are much worse, or that you are facing death? Or if you really want to recover, then you look at it in another way. Is this a good symptom? Does it show how much better I am? Does it not prove that I am really recovering?

Nothing misleads and disappoints us more than symptoms. We are poor judges of them and cannot tell where they lead and what they prove. In one person, a symptom may be very serious, which in another may be quite the reverse. It can prove an opposite signal in opposite states and different constitutions.

Therefore it is best to leave symptoms to your doctor and to turn your mind away from every temptation to consider the results and probabilities. It is best to abstain from the common but damaging habit of taking your temperature or pulse continually and trying to discern things from the results.

Just take the present moment as it comes. Look at its circumstances as the very best for you, because they are those in which God has placed you and which He could and would change, if He saw that other circumstances would be better for you.

Your present pain, He allowed. Each trial is His messenger. Do not say, *"Lord, we do not know where you are going. How can we know the way?"* (John 14:5) for His gracious answer now, and always, is: *"What is that to you? You follow me!"* (John 21:22).

PART III - DUTIES AND RESPONSIBILITIES OF ILLNESS

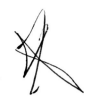

3.1 Contentment

There are few things through which the sick are more tempted by, than by discontent[56]. There are few aspects in which discontent does not offer itself manifest itself to those who are ill.

There is discontent with one's lot, with one's circumstances, with one's friends, with one's suffering and with everything which surrounds one. It manifests itself either in complaining or murmuring against God or in dissatisfaction. It may show itself in being difficult to please, in seeking to get one's circumstances altered or in a state of utter selfishness which refuses to take an interest in other people or in anything beyond itself. It may manifest itself in claiming that one's situation is "the hardest, the most trying and the least understood by others". It may be shown in constantly calling the attention of others to ourselves and to our trials or in a craving for sympathy. All these things mark discontent.

Discontent is seen in our face and expression, as well as in the voice. A person's manner can betray it. Some people want it to be seen in the hope that they get more sympathy,

---

[56]*"But godliness with contentment is great gain"* (1 Timothy 6:6). A state of mind in which one's desires are confined to his lot whatever it may be (1 Timothy 6:6; 2 Corinthians 9:8). It is opposed to envy (James 3:16), avarice (Hebrews 13:5), ambition (Proverbs 13:10), anxiety (Matthew 6:25, 34), and complaining (1 Corinthians 10:10). Contentment arises from the inward disposition, and is the offspring of humility and of an intelligent consideration of the rectitude and benign aspect of divine providence (Psalm 96:1, 2; 145), the greatness of the divine promises (2 Peter 1:4) and our own unworthiness (Genesis 32:10); as well as from the view the gospel opens up to us of rest and peace in eternity (Romans 5:2) (from The Easton Bible Dictionary under Contentment).

and they make no effort to hide it. They warm to people who will listen to their complaining and they count everyone else "hard-hearted".

But is there no sin in discontent? There is certainly misery. Discontented spirits are ever *"seeking rest, but finding none"* (Matthew 12:43). When in company with others, those who are discontented crave for attention and sympathy. When they are alone, they turn inward upon themselves, wearied, disappointed and more hopeless than ever. They brood over their distresses, never know the blessing of peace.

There is only one remedy for discontent. That remedy lies within the reach of every sick person but each must apply it, him or herself and must earnestly cry out to God to give the strength and the courage, the patience and the perseverance, to apply it faithfully and constantly.

The remedy is contentment. There are many ingredients in it:

- to see and to believe that you are discontented
- to feel the greatness of the sin of discontent
- not to allow yourself any excuse or evasion e.g. not to say, "Perhaps I am rather discontented sometimes but then I have so much to make me so"
- to hide nothing from yourself about it, but simply to recognise that "I am discontented"
- to consider it your duty to fight against discontent, beginning with some small thing which is the most obvious to you
- remember that this is a "holy war" that you are beginning and one which you cannot fight alone and in which you must daily ask for the help of God
- do not be downhearted if you make very slow progress and find the difficulties increase rather than diminish.

Sickness: its Trials and Blessings

"*The battle is not yours, but God's*" (2 Chronicles 20:15).

Your friends have been far more patient with you than you have given them credit for. You have wearied them frequently. They have really tried to please you, to make you happy and failed to do so. You have complained about them and, eventually after many hard thoughts about them, you have become estranged from them.

No wonder you are unhappy! Your state is a very painful one and calls for true pity. Have you asked yourself whether there may not be something in you, which prevents you from receiving what you crave and which seems to shut up and shut out, the love of friends and to leave you (as you suppose) a sad and isolated being?

You think your lot a hard one, perhaps even unlike the lot of anyone else? But who placed you in that lot? Is it not written "*The lot is cast into the lap, but its every decision is from the Lord*" (Proverbs 16:33)?

Have you ever thought that every aspect of your situation is under God's control? If so, have you any right to complain about it? Ask yourself honestly : are there any crosses which I complain about that I have brought upon myself? Do you never say, or make it appear that you should like something and then complain afterwards about it and say that it tired or annoyed you?

If you can answer "No" you are fortunate. But if your conscience answers "Yes: it is true", then this shows discontent which is an unwillingness to be satisfied.

Do you self-pityingly complain to everyone or to those home you confide in, until your whole mind is full of your grievances and you can think of nothing else when you are alone?

Are your prayers even complaining prayers, perhaps often rather about the failures of others, than than about your

169

own? Truly, this is one of the surest indications of a discontented heart.

Do you never, when you are alone, list all the frustrations & irritations of your circumstances? Do you think of all the things that could be better, like the characters of your friends, and even of your nearest kin, until you have an entirely exaggerated view of everyone and of every circumstance? Do you afterwards, perhaps unintentionally, distort things, in your own mind, and to others, in a distorted way, giving a false gloss and unreal colouring to them?

A faithful and sincere answer to these questions will teach you how truly to reply to the question. So is there no sin in discontent?

There are three sins in discontent:

- sin towards God
- sin towards your neighbour
- sin towards yourself.

Sin towards God

God has placed you where you are. He has chosen for you your friends, your home, your trials, your blessings, your pains, your pleasures and everything that makes up your situation.

He has chosen them because they are the best for you because those are the things which will the most quickly perfect you and make you most like Himself.

Sin towards your neighbour

He could change them in one moment but doing so, He would not prove His love. Your discontent has given you hard thoughts of God. Or at least they have proved obstacles to love, obstacles to anything but the kind of love which selects a few to care for, in other words, only those who meet your wishes, and then rejects the rest. Read 1 Corinthians 13 and test yourself by it.

Sin against yourself

You have by discontent, cut yourself out from the enjoyment of all the blessings and helps and comforts with which God has surrounded you ~~with~~. You have kept yourself from peace, rest, quietness and you have isolated yourself. If your sight had been cleansed, you would have seen the bright and blessed things around you which were things to be thankful to God for and to rejoice in. If your ears had not been deaf, you would have heard loving voices and they would have touched your heart and made it rejoice and sing. In not being like this, you have sinned against faith, hope, and charity. You have not trusted God. You have not *"hoped all things, believed all things, endured all things"* (1 Corinthians 13:7) nor persevered in loving, even when you imagined that no love was being given to you. This would have been the *"fulfilment of the law"* (Romans 13:10) and would have undoubtedly brought you blessing.

It is not too late to begin to lead a new life. Do not deny that it is impossible. The "God of Hope" can give you hope to enter into His Way. The "God of Love" will lead you, step by step, until you are *"changed into the same image"* (2 Corinthians 3:18). Only be serious about it. Be determined and steadfast. Do not give up over little things.

First, ask God to show you the sin in your heart and what a real, living thing it is. You never can be seriously a Christian, until you have done this. Do not ask once but again and again. Do not stop asking, even when you imagine that you are improving. Start by deciding that you will never complain about a certain topic again. Or if, as is most likely, you forget your resolution, then confess it before God immediately and humbly ask His forgiveness.

Next, try to find some bright spot, something to be satisfied with and even to be thankful for. Continue gradually as your spirit grows stronger, to add to the topics on which you do not complain and those for which you can be thankful.

In this way, very slowly, your heart, which was once dark and gloomy, will become bright and happy. The discontented thoughts about your friends will change into wonder at their love and kindness, until your heart seems to expand and glow. Your spirit will rejoice.

The entire world will change its appearance. You will wonder why the 'eyes' of your mind were formerly so blind and your heart so cold and loveless. This is no ideal picture, but the truth. Try it to see if it is genuine, make it your own. Then you who now "*go forth weeping, shall doubtless come again rejoicing, bringing your sheaves with you*" (Psalms 127:6).

Scripture says, *"Now there is great gain in godliness with contentment"* (1 Timothy 6:6). It does not merely say "*godliness is great gain*". Does this account for the fact that many so-called godly people are so discontented? The Scriptures tell us, "*But if we have food and clothing, with these we will be content*" (1 Timothy 6:18). But how have we obeyed this command? Another verse of Scripture says, *"You shall not covet"* (Exodus 20:17), and, *"Keep your life free from love of money and be content with what you have, for he has said, I will never leave you nor forsake you"* (Hebrews 13:5).

Is discontent with any aspect of our situation close to covetousness? *"Covetousness which is idolatry"* (Colossians 3:5). It may be idolatry of the self, or of any other form of idolatry. *"And do you seek great things for yourself? Seek them not, for behold, I am bringing disaster upon all flesh, declares the Lord. But I will give you your life as a prize of war in all places to which you may go"* (Jeremiah 45:5). *"Give us this day our daily bread"* (Matthew 6:11 AV).

Sickness: its Trials and Blessings

If you are discontented with your lot, in any detail, be sure, you are finding fault with the will of God and doubting His love for you. If this is so, how much we sin. In fact, we daily sin. We have "*grieved the Holy Spirit*" (Ephesians 4:30). Let us set out minds on contentment.

To show our gratitude for His gifts is the best thing we can do for Him, for "*As for the rich in this present age, charge them not to be haughty, nor to set their hopes on the uncertainty of riches, but on God, who richly provides us with everything to enjoy*" (1 Timothy 6:17).

Contentment is perfect rest, and perfect peace. It asks for nothing, seeks for nothing, hopes for nothing, wishes nothing, but what God gives. It ceases to see how its condition can be bettered, knowing that what God has willed must be perfect. Contentment does not ask to see the reason why God does one thing or another or why He withholds things which look like blessings. With open hands, it receives all His good gifts and thanks Him for His love and care.

Contentment does not look on into the future with dread but knows that God will provide. It has no wants and no cares, except to know Him more and to love Him better.

This state is the duty of every believer and especially of those who are called to constant temptations to sin against contentment, in sickness. God does not make anything our duty unless it is possible to attain it, unless it is for our highest good and unless He gives us the strength to perform what He requires of us.

So let us truly understand what contentment means and seek it in our hearts: "*O Lord, my heart is not lifted up; my eyes are not raised too high; I do not occupy myself with things too great and too marvellous for me. But I have calmed and quieted my soul, like a weaned child with its mother; like a weaned child is my soul within me. O Israel, hope in the LORD from this time forth and for evermore*" (Psalms 131).

"O Israel, hope in the Lord! For with the Lord there is steadfast love, and with him is plentiful redemption. And he will redeem Israel from all his iniquities" (Psalms 130: 7, 8).

3.2 Sympathy

Sympathy[57] especially should be developed in us by illness.

No one who is sick has truly understood the lesson that it was designed to teach, until he or she has learnt sympathy. They may deeply feel their deficiencies in sympathy, for we are all by nature, hard and lacking in sympathy.

Human beings are very slow to learn true sympathy. It is very easy to sympathise with some people, people who suit our taste, and with those trials which are exactly like our own. But this is actually a form of self-love and selfishness. In sympathising with them, we seem, as it were, to sympathise with ourselves. We never forget the relation of their trials to our own. Thoughts of self-pity underlie our own sympathy. In fact, sickness, wrongly received, increases selfishness infinitely. But sickness, rightly received, gradually casts out the unclean spirit, *"whose name is Legion"* (Mark 5:9).

Sympathy is not natural to us. It can only be given to us by our sympathising High Priest as He was *"perfected through suffering"* (Hebrew 2:10) and so He perfects us. Avoid saying, with sorrow of heart, "I have no sympathy. My besetting sin has been to sympathise only with a few people and from the many I have always been tempted to turn away, a sin which I have too little resisted. There is something in that person's manner which I cannot be attracted to, and we seem to have few, if any, points in common".

Instead show sympathy if you want to receive it. Create the 'atmosphere' and you will inhale it also. Sympathy is not a natural gift, though a few natures may be so endowed with

---

[57] Sympathy may be defined as kindness toward someone who suffers; pity; commiseration; compassion.

it as to shadow forth the full reality which can only be obtained by living with Him who is perfect sympathy and through deeply thinking of that living water that flows from His pierced side. It is all in vain to seek for the gift of sympathy in ourselves as it is not there. We must grow to develop it and the best way is to feel that we are utterly without it. In this way, we are driven to ask it of Him who *"gives generously to all without reproach, and it will be given him"* (James 1:5).

The way to grow in sympathy is to seek for increase of charity[58] or Christian love. The essence of sympathy is charity. No one without true charity can lack godly sympathy. He who was perfect love had perfect sympathy. The more we are conformed to the image of perfect love, the more we really understand and seek to practice St. Paul's description of charity ("love" in 1 Corinthians 13), the truer, the more abiding, the deeper will be our sympathy.

Sympathy is not a gift which once obtained will never fail or diminish. It is only by dwelling in the God of Love and of sympathy that we can shadow forth His love and His sympathy. It must be daily and hourly renewed and flow into our hearts, straight from Him. If we are convinced that we do not understand the wants or the trials of another, we must ask Him to interpret them to us or else to give us the words to speak, making us merely the channels of His grace.

There is another sense in which sympathy may be cultivated. We must constantly exercise sympathy, and not refuse it to anyone. We may resolve at all times to show interest in other people. They may come and tell us things which seem to us superficial trifles. We may be tempted to scoff at such a slight wound or to tell them this thing is of no importance. But bear in mind that nothing is a trifle which either tests another person or affects their welfare. Also, if we treat their test lightly, this person may be secretly hurt. They will not

---

[58] Charity, in this context, is another word for active love.

expect to receive sympathy for some greater wound and withhold the details from us. In this way, from the want of a little act of self-denial, we may have prevented ourselves from the delight and blessing of really helping them when we gladly would have done so.

Sick people should give everyone with whom they meet, a cause to feel that in any trouble, great or small, they will always find ready sympathy and a kind reception, never to be turned away. They must give cause to others to feel that they will be met with the greatest kindness, consideration, and encouragement. To do this requires continual self-denial both in body and the mind.

You may be particularly concentrating on some activity. If it is interrupted, try to avoid showing that you have been interrupted or that it is an inconvenience or annoyance to you. You may be trying to rest, but if a real demand for sympathy or help comes, do not refuse to meet it. You may be feeling peculiarly worn out in body and in spirit, but consider Him who said, when He was weary and hungry, *"My food is to do the will of him who sent me and to accomplish his work"* (John 4:34).

You may have been feeling worn out and are vainly seeking that quietness and calmness of spirit which has been taken from you by continued strain. You seem to have been attending to the claims of others all day. You have just laid down to rest and rejoiced in the comfort, when some new call upon your strength comes.

If it clearly is a call, do not turn away from it from it, but give ready, tender and loving sympathy. You will be rewarded for your self-denial if not now, then in Eternity, where all those acts which you may have long since forgotten will meet you again and where every tear of true compassion that you have shed will be remembered by Him who has commanded you to *"weep with those who weep"* (Romans 12:15). In Heaven, every smile by which you have cheered another person, every loving word, every sympathizing look, every pressure of the hand which touched a mourner's heart will be remembered. For there, Joy will meet you for every time that you have rejoiced with them that rejoice or have gladdened someone's heart, by your glowing or hearty participation in what has gladdened them.

Be assured that this shall be, because to show sympathy is to "walk in the blessed steps of Christ's most holy life"[59]. The tears which He shed on earth are 'guarantees', foreshadowing those which He sheds with us, day by day. And He would not have bidden us to "weep with them that weep" unless He had set us the example.

We never weep even in spirit, but He weeps with us. Be thankful, then, if He calls you thus to walk with Him. Often, the effort will be very great. You feel that your room is made the focus where all the troubles of the world meet. Sometimes, it is very wearying to you and you are tempted to wish it otherwise and to wonder why you have these additions to your burdens?

Rather rejoice that you are permitted to follow in His steps who never turned anyone away. He, when He was on earth called His disciples to come "*apart into a desert place and rest awhile; for there were many coming and going, and they had no leisure so much as to eat*" (Mark 6:31). When the people saw Him and followed Him, instead of turning them away because He and His disciples wanted rest, "*He was moved with compassion towards them, because they were as sheep having no shepherd, and He began to teach them many things*".

"*You go, and do likewise*" (Luke 10:37).

Remember, too, that there is encouragement in the fact that your friends bring their little troubles and anxieties to you. It is not the mere fact of your being "a fixed spot" in the

---
[59] a Collect.

Sickness: its Trials and Blessings

world and always to be found. It is this that causes them to do so. They would not continue to bring them if they found no sympathy from you and no understanding of their needs. Rejoice, then, to be made like your Lord and Master, for though you cannot go about doing good, you can lie still and let your friends come to you and attempt to do them good.

Do not imagine that you ought to show sympathy just in great spiritual trials and troubles, in all spiritual things, but not in temporal things. Let your sympathy be universal. You may be asked to decide between two colours, to advise on some article of clothing, to look at some book which may not interest you. The manner of your doing so for all you know, may affect the whole life of the person who asks you for advice. They may be struck with the readiness of your sympathy in a trifling thing which does not really interest you and it may draw them to you. It may make them feel afterwards, when some heavy trials come, that you, at least, could sympathize with them and they may turn to you. Then you may be permitted to offer them sympathy, in a really deep issue.

Try also to cultivate a sympathizing approach. Let there be sympathy in your voice, your tone and in your manner. Let nothing contradict your words. Kind words may be said often without it, but they fail to go to the heart.

But a word said with real tenderness and feeling may heal and soothe to an extent which we cannot evaluate in this life. This kind of discipline is a wonderful cure for that exacting spirit by which so many, and especially sick persons, are injured and distressed.

Never seek sympathy from others. *"Give, and it will be given to you. Good measure, pressed down, shaken together, running over, will be put into your lap. For with the measure you use it will be measured back to you"* (Luke 6:38). Give and you will surely receive it again, in far greater measure than you ever gave it, if not from those to whom you gave it, if not even from any friends on earth, yet from He who has said, *"Truly, I say to you, as you did not do it to one of the least of these, you did not do it to me"* (Matthew 25:45). He will give you a deeper and deeper knowledge and realisation of His own sympathy which "passes knowledge[60]".

3.2 Patience

The chronically sick need patience and patience of many kinds. Patience in bearing pain, patience in bearing all the deprivations caused by sickness and in bearing its many and accumulated trials. The patient needs patience to bear with those around him or her, with their sins, negligence and ignorance, and with all the misunderstandings and obtuseness. Someone ill needs patience to bear with their own circumstances in life, with their own peculiar lot. They need patience to wait for the *"appointed time until his change come"* (Job 14:14 AV).

It is indeed true that, *"You have need of patience"* (Hebrews 10:36 AV). The need seems to grow more and more intense, as time goes on. At times the difficulty of being patient may seem to decrease but then, again, it will soon become as difficult as before. At times, all the causes for impatience seem to gather strength at once and one's nerves seem completely shattered. Everything drains you. You see cause for impatience where you never did before, yet you feel utterly without patience and as if these words applied to you: *"Woe to them that have lost patience, and that have forsaken the right ways, and have gone aside into crooked ways"* (Ecclesiastes 2:16).

Sometimes the loss of patience is very sudden. You may seem, even to yourself, patient and quiet, when suddenly a fierce temptation to impatience may arise and overcome you

---
[60]Ephesians 3:19 "...and to know the love of Christ that surpasses knowledge, that you may be filled with all the fullness of God".

when you are quite unprepared. The impulse is momentary but the suffering involved in overcoming it and the sorrow of heart that you have been betrayed into sin will remain long with you and take from you confidence. You will feel as if it is hopeless to ever expect to become habitually patient, resting in patience.

Perhaps, in this case, as with sympathy, we tend to look on patience as a natural gift, a thing belonging to some people, while others are completely bereft of it. We speak of one or another person having a "patient character". Some people certainly have more natural patience than others, but it is unlikely that it will stand them well in a time of deep need or of sore conflict. Then it will be found that: *"The bed is too short to stretch oneself on, and the covering too narrow to wrap oneself in"* (Isaiah 28:20). Patient character will stand no such test.

In a short illness, the calls for patience are comparatively few. It is when the weary days continue, one after another, bringing their own petty trials hidden to bystanders, that its full need is felt. It is then that they who have been considered or who have considered themselves 'patient', know what a false reputation they had and what a false foundation they were living on. Now all the "gloss" has gone and they see themselves "*wretched, pitiable, poor, blind, and naked*" (Revelations 3:17).

In the past, you may have wondered why the Church prayed for all sufferers, that "they may have patience in their sufferings[61]". You may have thought that 'comfort' was the better and a more necessary thing to pray for them. Now, you understand what a knowledge of your current need was shown in that prayer. It is not comfort that you crave for, now, though you are very thankful to receive it when your Father

---

[61]Refer to James 5:10 "As an example of suffering and patience, brothers, take the prophets who spoke in the name of the Lord".

in Heaven sees fit to give it but, patience, or you cannot go on your weary way for another hour.

You sometimes feel secretly ashamed when a friend speaks of your patience. Patience! You who are in continual conflict with impatience and whose life is one struggle with it. You who seem to yourself for ever failing to hold your temper; whose tears and remorse could often witness how little you think that you have patience; you who groan before "*the God of patience*" (Romans 15:5), asking Him to make you like-minded with Himself.

At times, you almost think that people are mocking you and it makes you secretly angry. But there is encouragement in the words, because as deeply as you may have been aware of the inward conflict, you have reason to believe, if they are truthful and sincere friends, that your struggle has, by the grace of God been hidden from all eyes, but His. You have not been permitted to let it break out in deed or word. And so you "*thank God and take courage*" (Acts 28:15 AV).

It often happens that the long discipline of sickness and suffering is a gift to impetuous, impatient or over-active spirits. To them, of course, their natural impatience is like a constant fuel to the fire which burns within them and this discipline will be a very sore trial. If this is your case, remember that "*greater is He that is for you, than all they that are against you*", that "*the battle is not yours, but God's*" (2 Chronicles 20:15) and you "*in all these things will be more than conquerors through him who loved us*" (Romans 8:37). "*Suffering produces endurance*" (Romans 5:3).

A quiet, calm frame of mind, fixing itself on God, is the foundation of patience. In "*quietness and confidence shall be your strength*" (Isaiah 30:15 AV) which is also expressed by the words "*By your endurance you will gain your lives*" (Luke 21:19).

Sickness: its Trials and Blessings

Stillness produces patience. But we must first get into the right 'posture' before we can remain in it. What is patience but remaining in the posture of stillness? You will say, "How difficult this is!" Yes, it is. Should we say that it is 'impossible'? It would be, if it were not for the God of patience, who is our refuge. Therefore we can say, "*Why should I fear in times of trouble, when the iniquity of those who cheat me, surrounds me*" (Psalms 49:5).

We have no patience. Let us be clear about that. We must seek somewhere this thing which we so absolutely need. We have not far to go, for "*he is actually not far from each one of us*" (Acts 17:27) and He is "the God of patience". We need not ask Him to give it to us because even His own best gifts would soon perish in our keeping. Besides, we should soon grow proud of it, if we thought that patience were our own and the offspring of our own hearts.

Let us, instead, ask Him to unite us more and more to Himself, to enable us to dwell in Him, so much that we live in Him, walk in Him and act in Him. To dwell in Him so much that we are not able to do anything on our own. Let us ask to dwell in Him so completely that we always feel His strength supporting and upholding us, that we are in His arms and can rest there with all our weight resting on Him. Let us ask to dwell in Him so that we always ask Him to be with us and in us when we speak, never to allow us to be so hurried in ourselves that we shall not find the leisure and quietness to turn to Him.

There is no other cure for impatience except in increasing our unity with Him. There are, however, things we can do to increase our chances of overcoming the problem, through Him:

> a) When you feel impatience coming on, if possible do not speak because if you do, the words which you say will give you great sorrow and inner conflict.

b) If it is necessary to speak, commend yourself first to God like this; "O God, make speed to save us" or, "O Lord, make haste to help us"; "Lord, save me" or "Lord, help me". Any prayerful words will do but just let them be an act of commending yourself to God. Then be strong and do not fear. Speak what is necessary.

c) Do not torment yourself about impatience and be constantly imagining that you are impatient, or it will but make you more so.

d) Do not accuse yourself of the sin of impatience in an exaggerated manner.

e) When you have shown impatience to any one, whether to a friend or to someone helping or supporting you, acknowledge it and distinctly say that you know what you did, that you were wrong and are sorry. Say it briefly and do not try to excuse yourself. It is a most useful habit and a real route to humility if practised properly, especially when the person concerned is in a less powerful position, than yourself. It is the only restitution that you can make to them and the example will be a blessing to them. It will show them also that you were aware of your wrongdoing and that you do not sin, without conscience or without true repentance.

f) Observe which things stress your patience most and if possible avoid them. But if you cannot, if they come in your daily routine, then especially watch out for those 'weak points' and be on your guard at all times against them. If any particular person makes you impatient, be especially on the watch when you are with them. If you know that they are coming, ask God to be with you and to strengthen your heart. If not, then look up to Him at the time, for help.

h) Do not expect to be exempt from impatience: you cannot be, while you are weak. "*No temptation has overtaken you that is not common to man. God is faithful, and he will not let you be tempted beyond your ability, but with the temptation he will also provide the way of escape, that you may be able to endure it*" (1 Corinthians 10:13).

i) Remember that although sickness is a special opportunity for the exercise of patience, it is a state in which all the deepest impatience of your nature is stirred up and is often greatly aggravated by drugs and medicines.

The great remedy is to "*Consider him who endured from sinners such hostility against himself, so that you may not grow weary or faint hearted. In your struggle against sin you have not yet resisted to the point of shedding your blood*" (Hebrews 12:3-4). "*For this light momentary affliction is preparing for us an eternal weight of glory beyond all comparison*" (2 Corinthians 4:17).

What more than His help do we need? What more would we ask? Now our trials scarcely seem 'light afflictions', but they do not seem so slight because we look at them alone. "*For the things that are seen are transient, but the things that are unseen are eternal*" (2 Corinthians 4:18). Instead, let us more often look at those "*things which are unseen and eternal*", and these present things will change their appearance.

Let us bear patiently even the greatest trial of our own patience, if it is going to reveal our sin to us. Then we shall be enabled, in the strength of God, to overcome it. The trial simply makes us hang upon Him and learn that "*without Him we can do nothing*" (John 15:5 AV). "*A little while*" and the temptations and provocations to impatience will all be ended.

Let us bear the temptations now while God lays these "crosses" upon us. Let Him follow His own way of humbling us, which is sometimes to permit us to sin before and against others, so that we may learn how weak we are in ourselves and that there is no safety for us but dwelling in the "God of patience."

In this way, we shall be "*strengthened with all power, according to His glorious might, for all endurance and patience with joy*" (Colossians 1:11). Let us ask Him to enable us to exemplify

- "*a quiet and composed patience*" without the tumult of troubled thoughts and discontented passions;
- a submissive resignation without reluctance, to His will, of rebellious murmurings;
- a patience of hope that does not sink under our burdens, nor is driven by physical or mental pain to mistrust His love, care or gracious promises;
- a thankful patience, that is aware of comforts and supports as well as of our sicknesses; that considers all present sufferings to be far less than we deserve and all past and present mercies to be infinitely more than we deserve.

Make us perfect, O Father! In this patience, let us wait upon His leisure and not be hasty. Let us wait on Him and not grow weary but instead bear everything in the comforting hope of His strength to support our present weakness, of His mercy to comfort us and to deliver us at last, either to a more healthy life, or to a happy death, through the mediation of Jesus Christ our Lord. Amen.

3.4 Submission

Those who have truly learned patience have been learning submission, at the same time. However, there is a difference between patience and submission. Patience is lying in a still posture before God, waiting on His commands and in His timing. Patience is the refraining from all effort, vehemence and eagerness, everything that would get in the way off, or run ahead of the leading of God.

Submission is the actual surrender of ourselves, our bodies, souls, spirits and wills into the hands of God, the giving up everything to Him. It is the practical saying of the heart that says, "You know better than I do and you choose better than I choose". It is an act in which we yield everything in our life to Him and an attitude in which we are pleased with what pleases Him.

But submission is very slow in growth. This is because it wholly opposes and resists nature. We have strong wills of our own and they strive fiercely with the will of God. Even our prayers are the expressions of our self-will. Even, if we will not dare to say the words, do we not often mean, "My will be done"?

We may passionately pray that this or that thing may be given to us, which, if it were granted, would make us miserable for the rest of our lives! You may have asked for some special gift and instead of its being given, you have received the very opposite.

You have asked for work, active work for the glory of God and the answer to your prayer has been this life-long sickness. You have asked for patience and a sickness has been sent, which especially brings out your impatience! Everything that you have asked for, seems answered by the opposite. You have been almost tempted to cease from making any requests, for not one, it seems to you, has been granted.

You think that if you had asked for bright things and worldly gifts, you would have understood it. But you asked for things that your inner heart did not crave. What a conflict of spirit follows. Everything frustrates and upsets you

Sickness: its Trials and Blessings

and you cannot understand it. You were not so rebellious before your illness. You did not always so dislike the ways of God. Moreover you thought that you had truly given yourself up to Him.

You are not mistaken in how you see Him working in your life. It is just because you had not given yourself up to Him that He answers you like this. He has taken you to be His own and He will have you, wholly, entirely, without any reservations, "for richer or poorer; for better or worse[62]".

You have offered yourself to Him and now you must accept His terms. He will have no rivals, for *"He is a jealous God"* (Exodus 20:5). He says, *"My son, give me your heart, and let your eyes observe my ways"* (Proverbs 23:26). If you do give it straight away, He will have the whole, undivided heart. *"The idols shall utterly pass away"* (Isaiah 2:18). He will "c*ast them to the moles and the bats*"(Isaiah 2:20)[63]. Do not be surprised to see them cast out. Do not wonder if He "*makes a whip of cords and he drives them all out*" (John 2:15) so that your heart may be a fit dwelling-place for Him, a "*temple of the Holy Spirit*" (1 Corinthians 6:19), the *"dwelling place for God by the Holy spirit"* (Ephesians 2:22).

Your heart needs a great purging and refining. The process will be very long. Yet it must be like this if you are to attain true submission. At first, it is all about struggle, one unceasing fight. There is a perpetual sense of combat, of having your will at variance with His. Then, gradually, it becomes less and less so. But then, again, your own will seems to gain the upper hand and a fierce struggle follows.

You say internally, "Will it always be like this?" No, it will not. You may wrestle until all your resources are *"out of*

---

[62]from the Marriage Service

[63]"In that day, mankind will cast away their idols of silver and their idols of gold, which they made for themselves to worship, to the moles and to the bats".

Sickness: its Trials and Blessings

joint[64]" and your sinews are strained. Go on! Wrestle until break of day: the morning will dawn soon. For He who fights in you, will win.

In the utmost sense of your own weakness, you will resign yourself totally to Him. From then on, there will be more of His will in you, than of your own, or, at least, you will love His will better and grow in love towards it, day by day, until you will draw back from all other choices. You will feel that He knows what is best for you, and that you know nothing.

Then, you will find that in yielding to His will, there is rest and, sooner or later, pleasure too. So you will prefer to yield to Him, walking in the dark without knowing where you are going, than to choose or act yourself, in what seems clear day light. You will have learned that, *"God is light, and in Him is no darkness at all"* (1 John 1:5). In fact, you are in your own will, in utter darkness, only having light, when you walk in "the Light."

Do not think it is all over done and the conflict is ended. Your course is decided on. In that general submission to Him, you will see no alteration, since the real bias of your will now is towards Him. But the "changes and chances of this mortal life[65]" will still affect you while you remain here on earth.

You may get quite used to one set of circumstances while another set may come along, test your self will all over again and renew the inner conflict. It may be that the change in circumstances, to outward observers, may seem a pleasant one. They may be frequently congratulating you on it, while to you it may be a very trying ordeal. They cannot understand your feelings. They think you are a little odd, even unaccountable or even ungrateful. You cannot explain

---

[64]"When the man saw that he did not prevail against Jacob, he touched his hip socket and Jacob's hip was put out of joint as he wrestled with him" (Genesis 32:25). The "man" here is the Second Person of the Trinity.

[65]Collect, Book of Common Prayer

it all to them satisfactorily, and generally you are better not to even try. They could not understand that all changes, even for the better, are very trying to most of the sick though some crave for change incessantly, and will not be satisfied without it. It may seem eccentricity in you, and perhaps it may involve many inner conflicts.

Or you may have new associations, new trials to get used to and new circumstances to adapt yourself to. Eventually, your circumstances may become more pleasant but changes are new and therefore a trial. But instead of receiving any of the sympathy which you naturally expect, you are thought difficult to please and wayward.

Sometimes you get a lot of sympathy for something which is comparatively trifling, which you really do not think much of. This is because at the same time, there is something very trying, which is wholly unnoticed by all your friends even though it is eating at your very heart's core.

You find this a special trial, this inequality of sympathy and commiseration, this lack of responsiveness in others. It is a peculiar test of submission because it involves receiving the offered sympathy, for which there seems no real reason, thankfully and cheerfully and involves accepting the lack of the sympathy which you feel is really called for and for which your spirit craves.

Do not get upset. The more your trials are unknown and unnoticed the more entirely they can be borne for, and to God. If you offer them all up to Him, you will have His sympathy, such as you never could have had it, even if human sympathy had intervened.

"May He remember all your offerings and regard with favour your burnt sacrifices!" (Psalms 20:3).

Let the patient offer up his will to God in this, as in all things, and he *"will by no means lose his reward"* (Matthew 10:42). *"Submit yourselves therefore to God"* (James 4:7).

Sickness: its Trials and Blessings

God has many ways of teaching submission. Often when you are lying in a state of almost lethargy, of complete fatigue which is quite unutterable, there is, in fact, much passing between God and your soul. Or rather, He is working all His works in you, for you are lying still, scarcely conscious of anything but extreme exhaustion, and all its attendant suffering.

In fact, He is bending your will, He is teaching you how to yield yourself up to Him, He is teaching you the utmost of your weakness that you may learn what is meant by *"the Lord God is an everlasting rock"* (Isaiah 26:3). He is giving you the very trying discipline of 'nothingness', in order that you may learn what you really are, in His sight. He Himself is crushing you. Therefore fear not, for *"a bruised reed he will not break, and a smouldering wick he will not quench"* (Matthew 12:20). He will not lay His hand upon you more heavily than is necessary in healing all the wounds of your soul.

The greatest help in achieving submission is to receive everything straight from God. Do not look at second causes. Never allow yourself that excuse. Do not look back to the beginning of your illness and think how it first came on, how it might, perhaps, have been avoided, how it might have been removed in its early stages, how circumstances have aggravated it and do so still. Your case has nothing to do with these things.

God sent your illness, from the first. God permitted the errors and oversights of your friends, if you are aware of any. God placed you where you now are, exactly in the very circumstances in which you find yourself. Whatever you find fault with, *"Who are you, O man, to answer back to God? Will what is moulded say to its moulder, Why have you made me like this?"* (Romans 9:20).

Always bear this in mind and never forget it. When you are tempted to murmur against God at some little circumstance,

Sickness: its Trials and Blessings

ask yourself "Who appointed this?" Could God have prevented this if He had not seen that it was necessary for you? So answer, "God sent this: it is the will of God". Do not say, "All this is very true in great things, but how can it be true in little things and they are the hardest to meet with submission?" Can anything which concerns you be "a little thing"? Can anything which stirs up evil in you, or tempts you be "a little thing"?

If *"the very hairs of your head are all numbered"* (Luke 12:7 AV), is there anything too small for your Father to notice? No, be assured that He well knows how hard the little things are to bear and it is because of that that He permits them, *"so that the tested genuineness of your faith, more precious than gold that perishes though it is tested by fire, may be found to result in praise and glory and honour at the revelation of Jesus Christ"* (1 Peter 1:7).

Each of these little circumstances, humbly and patiently borne and will conform you to the likeness of your Lord and Master.

The whole life of Jesus on earth was one continued crushing of His Will. Do we desire that it should be different with us? "He Himself went not up to joy, but first He suffered pain; He entered not into His glory before He was crucified[66]". In the same way, our way to eternal joy is to suffer here with Christ and our door to eternal life is to gladly die with Christ so that we may rise again from death and "dwell with Him in life everlasting" (from The Service for the Visitation of the Sick).

Cease from all struggle. Let Him fight for you. Lie still in Him. Do not tease yourself with action. Find perfect stillness and rest in all His ways because they are the ways of the God of Love. Ask no questions but just believe that, *"What I am doing, you do not understand now, but afterwards you*

---

[66] Collect for Fridays, Morning Prayer (Book of Common Prayer). Also quoted in the Service for the Visitation of the Sick

will understand" (John 13:7). Do not say, *"Lord, why can I not follow you now?"* (John 13:37) but give yourself up to Him to lead you and to guide you and to carry you where He will.

This is submission.

3.5 Hope

One of the most necessary graces for a sick person to cultivate is hope. *"For the moment all discipline seems painful rather than pleasant, but later it yields the peaceful fruit of righteousness to those who have been trained by it"* (Hebrews 12:11).

The bright and joyful things are all beyond you and the dark and dreary things surround you. You look around and asks, "Where is the bright blessing of health?" The depressing answer is "It is gone forever".

No, it is not gone forever. It is awaiting you where "*there shall be no more pain*" (Revelations 21:4) where you shall be "*without spot or wrinkle or any such thing, that she might be holy and without blemish*" (Ephesians 5:27). But you must "*hope for what we do not see, and wait for it with patience*" (Romans 8:25). Yet, a little, and *"He will transform our lowly body to be like his glorious body"* (Philippians 3:21). This blessing has not yet come but it is in the future and you must hope for it now. *"Now hope that is seen is not hope. For who hopes for what he sees?"* (Romans 8:24).

To some people perhaps, hope is natural. They hope for everything and always look to the bright side, expecting the happiest and best result. This temperament is probably given to only a few and even they to whom it is given, if they endure long years of sickness, find hope becoming less and less naturally. Illness seems to eat the very life away and to make everything joyless and flat.

Sickness: its Trials and Blessings

Yet no one needs hope more than the sick. It is a dreary thing to lose all hope. Job describes a weary and depressed state, when he says, "*My days are swifter than a weaver's shuttle and come to their end without hope*" (Job 7:6). Prophets Isaiah and Jeremiah speak of "*no hope*" (Isaiah 57:10; Jeremiah 2:25) as being a state of complete dreariness. St. Paul speaks of "*having no hope*" (Ephesians 2:12 AV) as a state of those who are left with nothing.

It is true that "*Hope deferred makes the heart sick, but a desire fulfilled is a tree of life*" (Proverbs 13:12). Some have thought that it is better not to hope at all, than to have the chance of hope being deferred. They have imagined that in this way they will be spared from trial. But surely this indicates continual aiming after some earthly thing and the failure to attain it, when and as we will. Is this not the way in which we grow sick at heart and weary of delay? But if hope is a heavenly grace, given by God Himself, isn't it a good and precious gift and one that we are to seek by prayer, which does not become weary?

We should remember too, that it is as possible to sin against hope, as to sin against charity. In order, therefore that we may not commit this sin, we must keenly and continually cultivate hope. The sick who are shut off, for the remainder of this present life from the bright things of this world, who are too ill to enjoy life, are surely not being asked to hope for recovery, or to hope for brighter days again on earth? No. No such lesson is proposed, but rather the lesson of learning to say, "Your will be done."

Even the sick will find it a blessed and a purifying exercise to try to hope and to continue hope as a discipline. Some seem to themselves in prison, shut off from all the joys of life. But they are "*prisoners of hope*" (Zechariah 9:12), for hope which is seen, is not hope. "*What a man sees he does not hope for*" (Romans 8:24). It is future blessing that these souls should be looking for. Therefore hope calls for patience. St. Paul speaks of the *"patience of hope"* (1 Thessalonians 1:3 AV) and *"that we through patience, might have hope"* (Romans 8:24). *"Patience works experience, and experience hope"* (Romans 5:4 AV). *"It is good that one should wait quietly for the salvation of the Lord"* (Lamentations 3:26). Since *"hope purifies"* (1 John 3:3) it must be a blessed grace. Again, *"we are saved by hope"* (Romans 8:24). So we are not to lie in the grave of hopelessness but to look forward to the *"joy that is set before us"* (Hebrews 12:2) for *"hope does not put us to shame"* (Romans 5:5).

Earthly hope will often disappoint us, but heavenly hope, hope in things that are in the future will never "make us ashamed". Hope can put gladness into our heart. We are told about *"the rejoicing of hope"* (Hebrews 3:6) and *"a lively hope"* (1 Peter 1:3), a living bright reality. Hope is not an empty thing, but the *"full assurance of hope"* (Hebrews 6:11), the living certainty that those bright blessings are ahead of us, *"forgetting what lies behind and straining forward to what lies ahead"* (Philippians 3:13). It is *"a sure and steadfast anchor of the soul, a hope that enters into the inner place behind the curtain"* (Hebrews 6:19). Hope guarantees all things for us and turns them into realities. Through hope we realise these truths and we are enabled to *"abound in hope"* (Romans 15:13). That which we are to hope for is "t*he hope which is laid up for you in heaven"* (Colossians 1:5) and hope brings heaven nearer. It makes Heaven no longer seem a future thing, but that into which *"we which have believed do enter"* (Hebrews 4:3) feebly and faintly, but still "in heart and mind we ascend."

Hope makes all things become realities, as if they were already given to us. We possess them now and they are ours, if *"we are Christ's, and Christ is God's"* (1 Corinthians 3:23). *"The ploughman should plough in hope and the thresher thresh in hope of sharing in the crop"* (1 Corinthians 9:10). So should we, even though the seed may very long be hidden in the ground, continue in hope. We plough in hope, now.

This is the ploughing time, the sowing time, the harrowing time. The harvest will surely come. *"Hope to the end"* (1 Peter 1:13) and "*yet a little while, and the coming one will come and will not delay*" (Hebrews 10:37). We must not merely hope for future blessings, but even now *"hope in God"* (Psalms 42:5). Our souls may be very faint, but let us say heartily, *"My soul longs for your salvation; I hope in your word"* (Psalms 119:81). *"I will hope continually and will praise you yet more and more"* (Psalms 71:14).

All earthly pleasures seem to be fading away. You see no relief or enjoyment anywhere. Your own lot is full of depression and suffering. You experience conflicts and trials in your family. You look out at the world and it seems full of agony. Where is hope?

Do not say hope is gone. Instead, say *"Hope in God"*. "*God is Light, and in Him is no darkness at all*" (1 John 1:5). God only remains while the world is fleeting, passing away, even while you look upon it. You cannot find hope in the world. "*The hope of the righteous brings joy, but the expectation of the wicked will perish*" (Proverbs 10:28) because the Lord is the hope of the former. *"Happy is he whose hope is in the Lord his God"* (Psalms 146:5 AV). *"The Lord will be the hope of His people"* (Joel 3:16). If earthly things fail you "*we do not want you to be uninformed, brothers, that you may not grieve as others do who have no hope"* (1 Thessalonians 4:13)."

If your friends die, believe that if your friendship was 'in God', you will surely meet them in His presence and He has simply "sent on your treasures" so that they might be kept safely for you, and so that you may be drawn in spirit to Eternity. A little while and you will find that your hope was no delusion but a reality and that the "*hope laid up for you in heaven*" (Colossians 1:5) is kept by the God of Hope.

Ask God to give you hope, day by day, so *"that you may abound in hope"* (Romans 15:13) and thus glorify Him, like Abraham, who *"hoped against hope"* (Romans 4:18 AV) when everything seemed against him. Yet because God had promised, therefore he still hoped. Abraham's hope was so steadfast that at the command of God, he was ready to sacrifice his hope : his only son. In the same way, we must we learn to give up all our best earthly hopes and sacrifice them if God calls us to, knowing that we have *"a hope laid up for us in Heaven"* (Colossians 1:5).

While we remain on earth, let us hope in God saying, *"Why are you cast down, O my soul, and why are you in turmoil within me? Hope in God; for I shall again praise him, my salvation and my God"* (Psalms 42:11).

"May the God of hope fill you with all joy and peace in believing, so that by the power of the Holy Spirit you may abound in hope" (Romans 15:13).

5.6 Cheerfulness

You cannot have true cheerfulness whilst you are fiercely struggling. It will not come until your heart is at rest and you have the inner peace to forget yourself. If you have a complaining spirit, you cannot have true cheerfulness as it will generally show itself in your face and voice. Some little fretfulness or restlessness in your tone will always betray it. Your cheerfulness is forced, not spontaneously coming from your heart, which it can only do when your heart is truly at rest in God. You need to be satisfied with His ways and wish no alteration in them. When this is truly the case, then your heart and mind will be liberated and you will be able to rejoice in spirit.

When you have ceased to be preoccupied with yourself, you will have time to consider others, to make them happy. You will seek to be a bright presence, cheering, healing and strengthening those around you, especially members of your own family. You will always seek to welcome them all brightly, cheerfully and courteously, whenever they visit you or come into your presence or room.

Even if you are feeling weary and exhausted, you will rouse yourself to say some kind word, or to give a smile of kindness. You will try to overcome that nervous feeling which so often makes you draw back from looking at people, makes you imagine that you would cry or laugh if you did, and that the fixing your eyes anywhere is almost impossible. You will earnestly endeavour to warmly greet people and not to only a chosen few only and to make everyone feel that they are welcome, even if their coming is an unwelcome interruption and seems an unfortunate one.

Take it as a trial, from which you may receive real blessing if you receive it cheerfully, patiently, and submissively without questioning. At any rate, do not show that their visit is inconvenient or that you wish them to leave. If you do, you will lose the personal blessing that you might have received, the relative one that you might have imparted.

Of course, there are times for every sick person, when they are really unable to see their friends, even the members of the own family. When this is the case, it may be explained very sensitively and made apparent that *"The spirit indeed is willing, but the flesh is weak"* (Matthew 26:41).

Do not meet people with dullness, coldness or lack of concern. For the time you are with people, give yourself to them, make their interests your interests, encourage them to speak of themselves and their affairs and do not lay your burdens upon them. The more you learn to bear the burdens of other people, the lighter your own will become.

You may say "This is a severe lesson". How can you, who have been lying alone for so long, pondering your many trials, difficulties and privations, make strained efforts on behalf of others, who have worn your body and your spirit?

Sickness: its Trials and Blessings

How can you, in a moment, lay aside all these burdens and meet others brightly and cheerfully, as if there were no pressure upon your own spirit?

To say that the effort is great would not be enough. It will not be attained by one or even by a few desultory efforts, but by a continued, persevering effort, made in and with God. You may have insurmountable difficulties, you may not succeed in your desires and you may often be met with a cold absent manner when you have made the greatest effort to meet your friends warmly and kindly. A sense of coldness come over your heart, painful and overpowering. But do not be discouraged. Persevere, and He whom you serve will crown your efforts ultimately with success and will make the effort decrease. Remember that it is written, "*the one who contributes, in generosity; ...the one who does acts of mercy, with cheerfulness; the one who does acts of mercy with cheerfulness*" (Romans 12:8).

All the pleasure of receiving mercy, sympathy, kindness is removed when it is offered cheerlessly and heartlessly, wearily or languidly. Perhaps by nature, you have no cheerfulness in your constitution or you never cultivated it. You thought it was a natural gift and that those who did not have it not were not responsible for their lack of it. You have learned to view it differently now and feel that it is a high Christian duty, one very difficult to attain, and therefore needing constant exercise.

At first you were without hope about it. You said that you could never be cheerful, that you had naturally depressed spirits and that illness had added to the depression. You said that it was unreasonable to expect that people ought to bring cheerfulness to you and to expect that you should be cheerful towards them. You say that you have had such a constant drain on your own spirits, that you need that your friends to come and renew them for you, bringing subjects of interest to you and to amuse your mind.

Sickness: its Trials and Blessings

You tried this approach and found it failing, completely, because it was always an uncertain and unsure ground of comfort. Besides, you were fitful and were not easy to please or amuse. Friends said and did the wrong thing, at a wrong time, until you made it a trial to your friends to come to see you. You saw that there must be something wrong and then the secret was revealed to you. You were depending wholly on fellow humans, trusting them to cheer you and not living independently of all earthly people and circumstances, living in God alone.

At first, the discovery was painful to you, devoid of all hope. But gradually you turned to "*the God of consolation*" (Romans 15:5) and asked Him to enable you to let "*others recognize that you have been with Jesus*" (Acts 4:13). Nor was this all. You learned to rest in Him, to be content, not to complain and soon, you were so freed from thoughts of yourself, that you were able to give your thoughts to others, to an extent, which at first, seemed to you impossible.

How many rewards you have already received, even though, as yet, you poorly perform the lesson. Even your health is better for it. Your mind has ceased to prey upon itself and to react on your body. Now you every advantage is given to remedies and you have the best hope of recovery. You have hours and days of gladness where you used to have misery and sighing. You find life a far more pleasant thing than you ever imagined it could become.

You have the joy of feeling that you can impart happiness to others and that you do not cast long shadows on them. You have innumerable interests to occupy you and to prevent your time from hanging wearily on your hands. You have a foretaste of that bright world to which we are hurrying where "*neither shall there be mourning, nor crying, nor pain any more, for the former things have passed away*" (Revelations 21:4). By cultivating this spirit, you will gradually learn completely to "*rejoice with them that do rejoice*" (Ro-

Sickness: its Trials and Blessings

mans 12:15 AV) so that their pleasures will become your own and you will have a true share in them.

Try often to plan pleasures for others, to consider their tastes. Then simply and without effort, propose what you think will meet their interests. In doing so, you may often have to deny yourself, to make some arrangements that will disturb your usual habits or will be an inconvenience to you. This will be very good for you, a wholesome discipline. Do not let it be "seen of men" as it would spoil their pleasure and would surely rob you of the blessing. Instead, show real hearty, unconstrained pleasure in everything which gladdens another person's heart.

Thoughts may indeed seem to cast long shadows on you, to speak to you of your captivity, to remind you of the days when you could have joined in with things and enjoyed them, as others do. But do not let these dark thoughts darken your face. Offer them to God alone, and ask Him to give you grace with your whole heart, to say, "Your will be done".

There is sometimes, a sort of turning away, an averted look, an audible sigh, when others are going out to enjoy themselves and you cannot go. This is not cheerfulness and must not be permitted in yourself. These things must be crucified. Let your heart go along with your friends, enjoy life with them. When they return, willingly and cheerfully, listen to everything they tell you. If they have been where you have never been, seen people you wished to see, but have been prevented from seeing, do not avoid hearing about them but hear everything, with true interest and you will feel as if you had been with them. In the joy of giving pleasure, you will receive a large measure yourself.

Seek to cultivate the habit of enjoyment. It is wonderful how it grows and strengthens. A flower may be brought to us, and we may carelessly accept it. We may perhaps put it in a vase of water, or we may look at it, smell it, have it by our side and enjoy it, finding much instruction in it. We may be cheered too by the kindness which brought it. So it is with everything else.

You know not what blessed influence on people who come to see you through cheerfulness who come to see you. They may be strong and healthy now, but sickness may come upon them too. The remembrance of your cheerful sick room may prevent them from dreading it, as much as they would have done, if their impressions of a sick room had been only those of gloom and sadness. They may be tempted to much complaining and discontent, but the remembrance of your cheerful face may be a rebuke to them, or it may lead them to wonder what it was that made you cheerful in the middle of so many trials. They may never give up their search until they have found *that "with Him is the well of life"* (Psalms 36:9 AV).

Children, too, may retain a sad or a bright impression of you all their lives. Therefore, as *"none of us lives to himself, and none of us dies to himself"* (Romans 14:7) let us seek to live to others, so that our lives may be a blessing to others, eternally.

Always remember that cheerfulness may not be natural to you and that you are bound to seek for it and to give yourself no rest until you are vigorously cultivating this great Christian duty. God alone can teach you how "cheerfully to accomplish those things which He would have done[67]". Strive earnestly to *"lay aside every weight, and sin which clings so closely, and let us run with endurance the race that is set before us"* (Hebrews 12:1), every hindrance to the great duty of cheerfulness.

Perhaps one of the greatest burdens is not living in the present, either but allowing your mind to dwell on past times and pleasures now gone, on blighted hopes and on purposes unfulfilled , which were stopped by sickness. There

---
[67]The Book of Common Prayer (Twentieth Sunday after Trinity)

is the thought of hindred employment, work taken from you and your whole self, changed and shattered. Or else, perhaps, you are living in the future, forming for yourself some dream of what you will do when you recover your health, how things will be with you, how you can renew all your past enjoyments and give them a brighter glow than they ever had before.

All this cannot fail to make you discontented with the present and will make your lot seem sadder. You can never be cheerful, until you feel that every one of the circumstances in which you now find yourself, you were placed in by the God of Love. That is your calling and you are to abide in it, as long as He pleases which is to say that you are to be *"stable and steadfast"* (Colossians 1:23) not seeking for, or desiring change[68].

5.7 Thanksgiving

Those who are really feeling and appearing cheerful will already have been prepared to join in thanksgiving.

The other duties of the sick, which are contentment, sympathy, patience, and cheerfulness, may be said to be "our duty towards our neighbour[69]", though each one has also much in it of our "duty towards God[70]". However, submission and thanksgiving are especially our "duty towards God". *To "give thanks to Him for all things"* (Ephesians 5:20) is in-

---

[68]It is not that one should not try to aid recovery since health is a blessing. Simply that one should disregard the 'present' in illness, in the erroneous belief that it has no worth or value. One can be nostalgic about some aspects of illness, such as intimacy with fellow sufferers and the rapidity of growth in faith.

[69]Jesus teaches that we have a 'duty of care' towards men, women, relatives, the marginalised, employees and children: "Love thy neighbour as thyself".

[70]Duties towards God is set out in the first four of the Ten Commandments

deed, a very difficult task. This is because it includes giving thanks for trials of every kind, for suffering and pain, for languor and weariness, for the thwarting of our will, for contradictions, reproaches, loneliness and for deprivations.

What a hard duty it is, most of which is learnt very slowly. Yet those who have learned submission will not find it a hard duty, for they will so entirely love everything that God wills and appoints for them, that they will see that each circumstance is the very best for them and one which they could not have been spared. This will be a foundation for thanksgiving. Afterwards, they will see that He gave them just what they would have chosen for themselves. In looking back, they will see the links of the chain and how wonderfully each fitted together in their lives, even if, at the time, there seemed to have no sense or unifying pattern. This belief enables them to praise Him and give thanks for everything, assured that just as it has been in the past, it will be in the future and that the God of Love will do all things well. Therefore, while He is doing each thing, we will see some cause for thanksgiving. At this moment the notes of praise are very feeble but they will swell more and more until, "with all the company of Heaven, we laud and magnify His glorious name[71]".

Do not distress yourself if thanksgiving seems so difficult a duty. It is foreign to your nature but it will grow easier and more delightful to you, in proportion to practice. Begin with thanking Him for a little thing and then go on, day by day, adding new topics to your subjects for praise. In this way, you will find their numbers grow wonderfully and, in the same proportion, your topics for complaining will decrease, until you see in everything some cause for thanksgiving.

If you cannot begin with anything positive, begin with something negative. If your whole lot seems filled with causes for discontent, there is still some trial that has not

---

[71]The Communion Liturgy

been appointed you and you can thank God for that being withheld from you. It is certain that the more you try to praise Him, the more you will see how your path and your lying down, are set around with His mercies and that the God of Love is always watching over you to do you good. In the same way, as the sense of your unworthiness deepens, you will find more and more reason for thanksgiving.

Say to yourself, "Such mercies have been given to me and I am so unworthy of them. God is forever showing His Love to me and yet how little I thank and praise Him for it. He is always giving me good gifts but I receive them as a right, as if I had a claim to them. How little I have praised Him until now. He has been giving me blessings, ever since I was born, and I have scarcely noticed them. I have often taken them for granted and as matters of course, and, sadly still more frequently, I have complained about His gifts and complained about His loving will. And yet He has not been wearied by me or ceased giving His gifts, because I was ungrateful".

The first sense of this deep thanklessness is the most humbling. But we must be made conscious of our sins before we are able to say, *"I will give thanks to you, O LORD, for though you were angry with me, your anger turned away, that you might comfort me"* (Isaiah 12:1). We may lose our supports and comforts as the bright things of life pass away, but when we have learned that the will of God is pure and perfect Love, without change or variation and that all His ways are loving to us, then we shall learn to say, *"Though the fig tree should not blossom, nor fruit be on the vines, the produce of the olive fail and the fields yield no food, the flock be cut off from the fold and there be no herd in the stalls, yet I will rejoice in the LORD; I will take joy in the God of my salvation."* (Habakkuk 3:17-18).

There must be faith, hope and love in true thanksgiving. We must believe in God and believe that He is Love and that all

Sickness: its Trials and Blessings

His ways towards us are true faithfulness. We must hope in God, for "*hope purifies*" (1 John 3:3) raises us above the earth, brings all future things near and makes us see future things as realities even now as belonging to us. There must be Love, for we must entirely love God and His will and love our neighbour in Him and for His sake. In this way, we have our souls at rest, free from discontent and from jarring thoughts which would distract us and prevent that purity of heart out of which thanksgiving flows.

We shall look at things which are unseen, not at those sad and oppressive things which are seen. We will thank God for those realities and find all the more cause for thanksgiving, by contrasting those with the things which are seen.

We will look rather at *"that body which shall be"* (1 Corinthians 15:37 AV) rather than at *"this vile body"* (Philippians 3:21 AV) and thank God for it. Instead of looking at the areas in which our fellow-creatures give us pain, we will look at their love and their kindness, until we are astonished at it and at our own blindness which could not see it before.

Instead of mourning over your deprivations, you will look with wonder at the innumerable gifts which have been given to you. Instead of looking at yourself as unknown and unnoticed, you will come to wonder that so many people, sometimes even people unknown to you, think about and minister to you.

Instead of mourning that not a tree is granted to you on which your weary eyes can rest, you will thank God that even streets do not shut out the sky and that you can still gaze on that and feel that it is the work of God. Instead of thinking of all your crosses, little and great, you will *"turn away your eyes from beholding vanity"* (Psalms 139:37 AV) and fix your eyes upon His Cross, which was so sharp and so painful, and which was borne for you.

What have you to liken to His Cross and Passion? The reviling of enemies, the failure of friends, even of the dearest, the ignominy, the betrayal, the scourging and finally, the Crucifixion. What have you to liken to these things? He and He alone, could only say, "Was ever grief like mine?"

The more we gaze upon His suffering, the more our hearts will answer, "Never was grief like yours". In this way, we shall learn that our troubles are "light afflictions". As our sense of sin deepens, our knowledge of His amazing love will deepen also, until we see on His side, nothing but Love, and on our side, nothing but deep ingratitude. You will wonder that "Your *eyes were kept from recognising him*" (Psalms 24:16) so that you never saw this reality before and have been living blindly, adding ingratitude to all your other sins.

When once you learnt to "*give thanks in all circumstances; for this is the will of God in Christ Jesus for you*" (1 Thessalonians 5:18) then the "*voice of thanksgiving will be heard in your dwelling*" (Psalms 118:15) and your heart will abound with thanksgiving. When we feel that we owe much to a fellow human being, how our hearts go out towards them in gratitude and love. What a pleasure it is to thank them and to recognize their kindness to us. The more undeserving we feel the more this will be the case. How much more, then, shall we feel this towards Him. In fact: "*Every good gift and every perfect gift is from above, coming down from the Father of lights with whom there is no variation or shadow due to change*" (James 1:17).

Thanksgiving is a blessed and holy exercise and it elevates the whole being. You desire to glorify God? The Psalmist says, *"The one who offers thanksgiving as his sacrifice glorifies me; to one who orders his way rightly I will show the salvation of God!"* (Psalms 50:23). If our hearts were tuned to praise, we should see innumerable mercies which we had never seen before, for thanking God. *"Oh give thanks to the*

Lord, for he is good, for his steadfast love endures forever! Some wandered in desert wastes, finding no way to a city to dwell in; hungry and thirsty, their soul fainted within them. Then they cried to the Lord in their trouble, and he delivered them from their distress" (Psalms 107:1, 4-6).

Thanksgiving is spoken of as a *"sacrifice well pleasing to God"* (Philippians 4:18 AV). It is a far higher offering than prayer. When we pray, we ask for things which we want or we lay out our own sorrows. It is, in one sense, a selfish act. We pray, in order to bring down blessings upon ourselves, but we praise, because our hearts overflow with love to God and we must tell Him about them. The only reward that we expect is the delight which thanksgiving brings to us. How purifying it must be to go beyond ourselves, to stop thinking of what is good in ourselves and to start to think how good He is. This flows out of pure love, and then the love goes back into our own hearts and warms them, revives and quickens them.

But remember that praise is a 'sacrifice', one that God expects us to offer and justly claims from us. We cannot choose but to offer it because if we do not, we "rob God". *"Will man rob God? Yet you are robbing me. But you say, 'How have we robbed you?' In your tithes and contributions"*. (Malachi 3:8). God says, *"Let them sacrifice the sacrifice of thanksgiving, and declare His works with rejoicing"* (Psalms 116:17 AV). *"Let Israel rejoice in Him that made him; let the children of Zion be joyful in their King"* (Psalms 149:2 AV). *"Rejoice in the Lord"* (Psalms 33:1). *"Rejoicing in hope"* and *"patient in tribulation"* (Romans 12:11 AV) are closely connected.

Let us therefore say, *"I will offer to you the sacrifice of thanksgiving and call on the name of the Lord"* (Psalms 116:17). *"I will sacrifice unto you with the voice of thanksgiving; I will pay that I have vowed"*.

We often ask, *"What shall I render to the Lord for all his benefits to me?"* (Psalms 116:12). It is this sacrifice of thanksgiving that He would have us render. We must offer it through our High Priest, because all our offerings need to be purged and offered up, purely for us. *"Through him then let us continually offer up a sacrifice of praise to God, that is, the fruit of lips that acknowledge his name"* (Hebrews 13:15).

3.8 To remember those in need and to help others[72]

God wills that you remember the poor. *"For the poor you always have with you, but you do not always have me"* (John 12:8). If you have a true and living sense of His love to yourself, if you feel that He has *"done marvellous things"* (Psalms 98:1) you will feel that the large family which our Lord has left here on earth which needs to be tended, fed, and cared for, ought to claim a very large portion of your love and thoughts. You will seek by whatever means you can, shut up as you are, to help, cheer and bless them.

There are many ways of doing so. If you are a member of a family and not its head, it is probable that the very heavy expenses of sickness will not fall upon you. In this case, your needs will be so much fewer than when you were going out and about in the world, so that you will be able to redeem a larger portion of this world's goods for the poor. You can either minister to them through others, through your family or through your pastor. Or, if you are well enough, you may have the delight of ministering to them with your own

---

[72]Priscilla Maurice had been well aware of all classes at Guys Hospital. London and in her will, she established a convalescent care home for impecunious women at Catherine House, St Leonards-on-Sea. According to The Times (1902) she founded this home, possibly diverting money from the sale of her books. From 1855 to 1902, nurses and medical care looked after two thousand needy and sick women in the 22 rooms. Priscilla Maurice, herself, prepared from her sick-bed a summarised version of her book on suffering intended for the poor, so that people without much money could also read what she wrote.

hands. You may be able to send for them, one at a time and give them what you think they most need, while inquiring into their shortages and becoming affectionately interested in all their concerns. This, if you are able to do it from time to time will be a great help to yourself, taking from you the lack of purpose, the loneliness of sickness and you will learn by this interaction how light your own trials and deprivations are. It will give you much cause for thanksgiving. You have a comfortable room, kind attendance, food to eat, heating and many other blessings. Others, perhaps, have only one small, dark, unwholesome room for everything, in which a large family may be shut up, in fever, with no other place but a hospital to go to. They have no fresh air, no fire (or only now and then) and no attendant. They are often without necessary food, clothing or bedding.

Let all your knowledge of trial draw out your deepest sympathies towards them. Let your knowledge of your blessings and your wonderful exemption from such trials, stir up in you the spirit of praise. Perhaps you may be able to make clothes for them or to provide for their being made? Are you able send food parcels or other comforts? If you are the head of a family, you can easily arrange to have many things spared and saved for them, even though your finances may be very limited and your financial outgoings heavy. The more we look for opportunities of helping the poor, the more will the power and the will increase. Ways will open which were unseen before.

In giving to the poor so much depends on the manner in which it is done. A sympathizing manner shows real care for them with only a few kind words. This will strike home to their hearts, however small the gift given, whereas some great gift may be given harshly, or with a lecture about lack of care with money. Advice on the need for economy may be given with it, which may take from the gift all its value and make them feel only how little the rich know of the real life

Sickness: its Trials and Blessings

wants of the poor, and how little they sympathize with them.

You, especially, who have had the discipline of sickness and its deprivations, should show tenderness and sympathy. If you cannot visit the poor yourself, or see them when they come to your house, you will interest your helpers in them and make them your givers of gifts. It will do them much good also and will be a link between them and the poor, and between you and them.

All your attempts to help the poor you will offer to God as your "*sacrifice of thanksgiving*" (Psalms 116:17 AV) and will do everything *"as for the Lord and not for men"* (Colossians 3:23). In the same way, you will endeavour to help everyone who comes to you in need, *"For God is not unjust so as to overlook your work and the love that you have shown for his name in serving the saints, as you still do"* (Hebrew 6.10). You will help them if you can with the assistance of money, work or advice which you have in your power to give. Nor will you do this the less if your work is wholly hidden and it should appear to be theirs alone. You will see how good this is for you and you will gladly and thankfully see others working and cheer them on their way, even though at times you may suffer from the pain of the contrast between your life and theirs.

You will seek also to interest yourself in all works of mercy fulfilled by those societies and charities which are really trying to do the work of God, in an orderly and humble manner. Everything, in which you can interest yourself, will open to you a fresh and a wider field of enjoyment. Everything that belongs to God and to furthering His work on earth should have the deepest interest for you. You should seek to let it become, increasingly, a part of yourself, your thoughts, your prayers and of your labours.

Part IV - THE BLESSINGS OF ILLNESS

The blessings of sickness are so closely connected with its trials. The danger of trying to look at them separately from each other is so great that throughout this book, blessings and trials have been interwoven. This chapter is intended merely to gather up some of the pieces that remain, so that nothing may be lost.

> "How precious to me are your thoughts, O God! How vast is the sum of them! If I would count them, they are more than the sand. I awake, and I am still with you. (Psalms 139:17,18).

Was illness a strange answer to your prayers, or so you thought, when it came? You had prayed for a chance to serve Him and yet God sent you sickness and laid you aside. He seemed to read all your prayers backwards and to answer you with their opposites.

Do not doubt but sincerely believe that your sickness is the very best answer to your prayers. It meets them and includes them all. In it, and by it, your works will be purified and (what a strange truth) you will, if you handle things correctly, learn in sickness to "desire life and love many days" (Psalms 34:12). You will learn to "joy in the gifts Heaven's bounty sends[73]" and to see everything shining in the brightness which the love of God sheds around upon everything. You will learn to love God's will so much that you will desire nothing but what He gives.

Right now there are great blessings in being laid aside in illness. Have you ever considered how many evil, foolish and destructive things you have been protected from, by your illness? How many over-reaching ambitions and excesses you not only might, but certainly *would* have succumbed to,

---

[73]Unattributed in the original but taken from the poem, "A Voice from Afar" by John Henry Newman.

which, by the mercy of God in sending you sickness, have been put out of your reach? Before your illness, for example, how keen were you on debate and controversy which was leading you astray? Hasn't sickness taught you to feel the lovelessness and restlessness of debate and how much it engrosses the thoughts and draws you away from vital divine truth?

Sick people want real living truths. They want food, not husks and the simpler the truth, the better. You know that God is Love and you want to be like Him. You do not want to be tempted to *"bite and devour one another"* (Galatians 5:15).

Before, you were feeding on husks. The Voice could have said, "*Let him alone*" (Luke 13:8) but instead it said, "*Return to Me*". *"Therefore, behold, I will allure her, and bring her into the wilderness, and speak tenderly to her"* (Hosea 2:3).

Think back and consider whether you had begun to care more for the outward visible signs of spiritual things, than for the inner things. But now you have been removed by sickness, from your idolatry of outward forms, so that you can see them at a distance. Now you see how much had been added to the essentials of spirituality by mere men and women, and by your own earthliness of heart. Now you see how little or much in those idolatrous forms was living, true and holy. You have been taken from hearing of penitence, in order to learn to be penitent. You have been taken from hearing that "Christians should love each other" to dwell more alone with Him who is Love, so that you may be changed into His image.

You have been laid aside in illness so that you may learn what His truth is with less confusion than you could learn it, while you were in Babel[74]. You have been brought into the

---

[74]The Biblical Babel (Genesis 11:1-9) was the city and tower in the land of Shinear where confusion of languages took place. A place or scene of noise and confusion; a confused mixture of sounds, voices or languages.

Sickness: its Trials and Blessings

presence of the truth where all masks and superficialities are gradually removed and the soul becomes more and more alone with God.

Perhaps, looking back, you once thought that you would make some great sacrifice, render some great service to God or separate yourself from the world? You despised domestic duties and thought them poor and worldly, not containing enough in them of spiritual sacrifice. But didn't you overlook the hourly and continual calls in them for real self-sacrifice, for renunciation of the will, for subduing your temper, for "forbearing one another in love" and for mortifying your pride and vanity, in self denial.

All those things were so close at hand that you could not see them because you were looking for a wider scope, something further afield. God heard your prayers and He answered them, not as you would have had them answered, but as He saw, in the best way.

God said, "*Do you seek great things for thyself? Seek them not*" (Jeremiah 45:5). He has also said, "You wish to make some great sacrifice and you shall have the desire of your heart. You shall sacrifice your will and lay that upon the altar". You could not be called upon to make a greater sacrifice, so make it willingly and cheerfully.

Can you see, now, all the distractions into which you would have enticed if you had be given health? Can you imagine all the worldly traps into which you would have fallen and all the dangers which you have escaped? Instead of complaining at sickness, loneliness and weariness, you should thank God for no mercy more fervently than for sickness.

Now that we have considered sickness with its many sorrows and trials and hidden sufferings, as well as its many blessings and mercies and comforts, don't you see that there is a wide field still open before you? Do you not see that the map of your life is not as diminished as you previously thought? Do you see that there is much work still, for you to do?

This work is real work, some of which you could not have done without sickness and none of which you could have done so well, without its discipline. You may, indeed, seem to yourself, and to others, to be doing much less than you used to do, and to be doing less than they expected, and still expect of you. But be assured that if you rightly receive your sickness, whatever work you do is done with so much more simplicity and sincerity and with so much purer motives than ever before, that what you do, having more of God in it and less of you in it, is far more precious in His sight and more valuable to those to whom it is directed.

You remember, no doubt, how much you did in time past, either to be seen by men, to please other people or to satisfy your restless, busy nature, which must always be working. Did you get pleasure in doing some great thing which would get you glory and recognition in the eyes of others? Now, how differently everything appears. You cannot, even if you wanted to, achieve this now.

Now can you see as never before, not only the intense pleasure of being permitted to work for God, in the least vainglorious things, which before you would have overlooked as too insignificant. Now you can see that there is nothing worth living for, except to glorify God.

If so, you have learned this through suffering. You have been brought to feel thankful to suffering, if it will only purify your motives and prevent you from *"doing the work of the Lord with slackness"* (Jeremiah 48:10). If sickness will only make you to look up to Him for your work day by day, and not choose it for yourself, nor complain because you have none, nor seek to do your own works.

If you are able to do this, then you will be able to look up to Him in the evening and thank Him for what He has enabled you to do, both for the work which He has given and the strength which He has given you with which to perform it. You will find it in your daily life, in your domestic chores and duties, those small and unimportant things which you used to overlook and think separate from the real service of God. You will find it in conversation with your friends, in the claims and call of those in need, in all that interests those with whom you are connected, and in all things which concern the Church of God.

You find your work, too, in struggling against all that is evil in yourself and in overcoming it, for your own sake and for the sake of fellow believers. Each victory that you obtain over the tempter, in His name and in the strength of the Lord, weakens the enemy's power over you, and over them, and gives the adversary a surer guarantee of being soon *"crushed under your feet"* (Romans 16:20) and under their feet too.

In every victory over the Enemy (the devil) or over your own selfishness and self-will, you find your appointed work and you fulfil it. Therefore, never entertain the weary, destructive thought that you have no work, nothing to do for God and are an isolated being. Wait a little, and "*there is a reward for your work*" (Jeremiah 31:16). *"Nothing is covered up that will not be revealed, or hidden that will not be known"* (Luke 12:2). You, and all mankind, will see that your sick bed was no hindrance to serving God and that you had work to do which you could not have done elsewhere. It was a work that was not part-time but filled up every hour of your day, whether you were seemingly busy, or lying almost in lethargy in a dark room, taking no notice of anything around you. Even there and then, you were working and God was by your side, appointing your work of suffering and measuring its measure and its nature. He was blessing it and you, and without that divine blessing of the suffering, the work which He has given to the Church would be imperfect.

In the most extreme exhaustion, in the utmost state of weariness or in the sharpness of pain, say to yourself, *"This is the will of God. It is His will that I should work for Him in this way. My portion is now this. In my flesh I am filling up what is lacking in Christ's afflictions for the sake of his body, that is, the Church"* (Colossians 1:24).

What a glorious work it is! What an honour to be called to it. How often in His sufferings here upon earth, Jesus was alone and no one saw what He endured, except His Father and our Father. Yet even then, He was fulfilling His ministry.

It is similar in your case, so do not give up. Your spirit may be growing very weary but simply strengthen your heart with the thought that you are suffering with and for Jesus Christ, and for His Body's sake, which is the Church.

When you are *"weary or faint hearted"* (Hebrews 12:3) think of what Jesus endured and of the high calling which it is to suffer with Him, to *"share his sufferings, becoming like him in his death"* (Philippians 3:10). He who has called you to this work and ministry is always alongside you. He said: *"I am with you always, to the end of the age"* (Matthew 28:20) sustaining, strengthening and cheering you.

You have one more blessing, which is that the Lord's Prayer is no longer a set formula for you or even merely words which you have pleasure in repeating. You want it now. It is necessary to your very survival. Every word of it has become charged with meaning, such as it never had before. Every sentence has a life-giving sound. Very often when you are unable to utter any words of your own or think any thought of your own, you can pray the Lord's Prayer in your heart and give thanks for it. You can give thanks in your extreme weakness and dependence, in your need of some person to rely on, of Someone to turn to in all your trials, sorrows, pains and perplexities. You can recall that there was One who knew them all and *"needed no one to bear witness about man, for he himself knew what was in man*" (John 2:25). He taught you to say, "*Our Father*" (Matthew 6:9) with a love and tenderness and confidence which you never knew before.

You rejoice to say "Our" because it tells you that you are a member of a family not a solitary being. When you say, "*Which art in Heaven*" then you are reminded of that "*there remains a Sabbath rest for the people of God*" (Hebrews 4:9), an "*inheritance that is imperishable, undefiled, and unfading, kept in heaven for you, who by God's power are being guarded through faith for a salvation ready to be revealed in the last time*" (1 Peter 1:4,5).

All the eager and restless desires of your heart for the glory of God and the advancement of His kingdom now seem to find their core and home in the words : "*Hallowed be Thy name, Thy kingdom come*". All your personal desires and wishes for yourself, your friends and all mankind are expressed in "*Thy will be done in earth, as it is in heaven*". Your daily need to be led and guided in work and strength, in your trials and your supports and in all your earthly needs are summed up in the petition, "*Give us this day our daily bread*". Your growing sense of sin, your knowledge of your ongoing "*sins, negligence, and ignorance*", your deep sense of lovelessness and your sufferings from it, make your whole heart say, "*Forgive us our trespasses, as we forgive them that trespass against us*". The ever-growing sense of temptation, of being "*sore hindered*" of "*the temptations of the world, the flesh, and the devil*", all these make your heart cry out, "*Lead us not into temptation, but deliver us from evil*". There is assurance in asking all these things, for "*Yours is the kingdom, the power, and the glory, forever and ever*". Therefore you can say, "Amen", so be it.

All things are in God's control. All that you have asked He can grant. You seem to begin each petition with, "*Our Father*" because those two words explain and run through the prayer. They give you the child-like confidence in asking which you so greatly need. "*Our Father*". Let those words blend themselves with every thought of your heart and with every action of your life. Surely *"Our Father"* would deal with us as with sons and would send us no needless suffering, no unnecessary correction. *"As a father shows compassion to his children, so the Lord shows compassion to those who fear him"* (Psalms 103:13). He will not give us into others' less able hands for our spiritual development. He Himself will develop us. *"I will discipline you in just measure, and I will by no means leave you unpunished"* (Jeremiah 46:28).

"Blessed are ye that weep" now, whether in persecution, bereavement, sickness, or fear. Every trial in the Christian life is an advance in your walk of faith. Every chastisement is sent to turn a new page in the Book of Life, to show you things within you which you did not see or know before, and things which afterwards shall be your calling. God is cleansing the power of your sight so that it may become intense and strong enough to bear His presence. That power of sight is Love, fervent and purifying Love, consuming every sin and purging every stain.

The more fervently you cling to Him by love, the clearer your vision of His beauty will grow. So welcome everything He sends, since by doing this, we may see Him on His Throne, where there is no more sin, where truth has no shadow and where unity and sanctity have no conflicts.

Welcome sorrow, trial, fear and the shadow of death, if only our sin be blotted out and our lot secure in the lowest room of Heaven, secure in the light of His face, before the Throne of His Beauty, in our eternal home and in our rest, forever.

Part V - MISCELLANEOUS

5.1 Reading the Scriptures

There is a casual kind of reading of the Holy Scriptures in which the sick often indulge. They are only able to read a little and therefore choose the portions they like the best and think will be the most comforting. In this way, they lose much of the message of the Bible by taking it in detached passages, instead of in context. By taking verses out of context, they often get a false idea of the meaning and many portions which would be very instructive to them they never read, choosing instead what their spiritual food should be, instead of having it given to them.

To use some systematic plan in Bible reading is a very great help in sickness and especially for those who are isolated from church[75]. It is pleasant to look to something to guide us and teach us and to tell us what to do. It prevents that vague feeling of wanting to know what is best to do, and how to read the Scriptures profitably. *"All Scripture is breathed out by God and profitable for teaching, for reproof, for correction, and for training in righteousness, that the man of God may be competent, equipped for every good work"* (2 Timothy 3:16-17).

Therefore, we should read the entire Bible in sickness. Otherwise we will miss something that is *"profitable for doctrine, for reproof, for correction, for instruction."* Reading detached chapters and verses does not meet our needs.

But can there be a better plan than one given by the Church? If we read the daily Lessons and Psalms, as far as our strength permits, we shall read the Old Testament once a year, the New Testament three times and the Psalms

---

[75]For example, a plan of daily reading offered by Scripture Union at: http://www.scriptureunion.org.uk/8.id

twelve times through. We will soon find how wonderfully each Lesson and each Psalm seems to bring something peculiarly fitted to our needs, at the right time every day. As we read them afresh, we shall discover this more and more and be able to recognise them as the portion given to us for our profit, not as a self-chosen selection.

We will have the happiness of not reading alone, but with *"many members of the one body"* (1 Corinthians 12:12 AV). This kind of reading of the Bible will not degenerate into a mere religious practice. In fact, it will become less so as you pursue it. Sick people do not need to fear falling into mere religious practices. They, perhaps most of all people, need them the most because they are deprived of so much that comes in the natural order of things to people in health. They are in great danger of growing too casual.

Often a husk may be thrown away as useless, not knowing that it contains a precious kernel. The husk may look like other husks, unsightly and irrelevant, but you cannot get at, or preserve the kernel without it. At any rate, do not throw away any practice, until you have examined it. In sickness, the only way of thoroughly testing it is by long and daily practice.

5.2 Sunday, the Lord's Day

Another subject of great trial to sick people are Sundays. Some feel this much more acutely than others. The lack of being able to attend public Church worship is, and ought to be, a great trial.

It is the great loss of meeting together, of having a place *"Where we supposed there was a place of prayer"* (Acts 16:13), of having a place where many are praying together, helping each other. It is the loss of a place where God is especially felt to be present and where a fixed time is appointed for prayer, the quietness of which cannot be broken by outward distractions and interruptions. It is the loss of the wonderful uplift in the sympathy of many people worshipping together since our sluggish souls need every help. It is also the loss of the voice of prayer which is a great assistance and keeps up our spiritual zeal. When praise is offered, the heart is lifted up like that of others and the "*voice of melody*" (Isaiah 51:3 AV) ascends.

In public worship, too, is the fulfilment of the great promise that may be claimed: *"Where two or three are gathered in my name, there am I among them"* (Matthew 18:20). There is the realisation that the Church is made of many members of one body, so that we can say, "I believe in the Holy Catholic Church, the communion of saints".

All these blessings of public worship are withheld from the sick[76]. The cheerful sound of the Church bells only reminds them that they cannot go up to the house of the Lord and the bells sound with painful sadness in their ears, if they have not learnt the lesson to "*rejoice with them that do rejoice*" (Romans 12:15 AV).

The extent to which absence from public worship negatively affects private devotions can only be known by those who have been for months or years, kept away from it. The habit, the fixedness, the place, are all lacking. It is a very difficult thing, day after day, to continue private devotions in the same unchanging place, with nothing outward to call you away from the world to call you to worship. In that very room, the same bed perhaps, you must carry on, everything. There you suffer your pains and sicknesses. There you see your friends. There you take your meals and transact all your worldly business. There you sleep and there everything which fills up your life is carried on.

---

[76]Today people laid aside by sickness can avail themselves of services broadcast through (Christian) radio and TV stations or through the internet.

Sickness: its Trials and Blessings

The outward help of being called to worship, of going to the house of God, of the companionship of worship, you never have now. You see others going and you sometimes wish that they would so connect you with their blessings and enjoyments as to say occasionally that they wish you could go with them. You would not wish them to say this all the time since then it would become a formality. Probably, it is their kindness that stops them, though they may be mistaken about what is best for you.

They think, often, that after so many months or years of confinement to the house you must be quite used to it and have long ago ceased to want to go to Church, feeling that it must not and cannot be. So they fear to stir up your longings again. Or they look on your being left at home as so completely a matter of course that they either forget you, or doubt that it can be any trial to you. Or else they suppose that you ought by now to be used to not going and that if you are not yet reconciled to it, you are in some way 'in the wrong'. Or they may think it a mere form to say words which imply impossibility. Or they cannot fully understand the measure and depth of the trial, because when, during any short illness they have been kept at home, it may be that they did not feel the effect that not going to worship produces on private devotion, in so short a time.

This also accounts for the fact, that when sick people begin to recover, after a long illness and are able to go to Church again, if they are prevented from going for one or more Sundays, they can display great disappointment. Their friends say, "I wonder that you should so much mind being kept at home for one or two Sundays, when you remember for how long you were prevented from going? Surely one Sunday cannot now be much of a privation to you?"

It is just *because* you have been shut up so long, that you feel the so acutely every obstacle now. You have learned the value of public worship. On top of this, you feel how insec-

Sickness: its Trials and Blessings

ure your hold on this blessing is and that you do not want to lose one opportunity, whilst you have it.

When your friends return from Church, you long to be connected with what they have been enjoying. How thankful you would feel to be voluntarily told about the sermon or even the text for the sermon. Sometimes you think that people ought at least to look happier and more cheerful on Sunday than on other days. You feel that their blessings are so great that it ought to be the brightest of days for them. It seems to be its very brightness that casts so dark a shadow on you.

Yet it seems to you that they often look wearier and seem more uncomfortable on that day, than on any other. You do not take into account that they have weary bodies which have been worn by the work of the week and that the very rest from that seems to bring weariness or listlessness. Nor do you take into account what a busy and occupied day Sunday generally is and how very little time they have to spare for you and that little left to them is given when they are tired by the labours and pleasures of the day. You forget that the spirit having been so much stretched during the week, is weary too.

There are, doubtless, some cases in which it would produce discontent, if it were said to a sick person: "I wish you could go with us". A few people might burst into tears, either those who have been ill for a short time and who have not as yet seen that they are wrong in indulging temptations to envy those who can go to Church. There are also those who encourage discontent in this and other ways, refusing to be comforted.

In the majority of cases, it would be found that the kindness of the words and the pleasant thoughts that others would like you to share in their pleasures would prove a great comfort. They would refresh and cheer weary spirits long after the words had been forgotten by the person who said them.

Their words seems half to take you to Church in spirit or, at any rate, give you a realisation of the Communion of Saints, in some minds, of course, more deeply than in others.

"I wish you could go with us". Internally you can say, "In spirit I can". The heart answers and already the feeling of isolation is gone. In its place is, "I believe in the Holy Catholic Church, the communion of saints[77]".

On the other hand, how often the sick person feels, as the last person goes to Church and shuts the door of the house, "If they cared that I should be with them, surely they would sometimes say so? How then can I hope that they will remember me there? I am cut off from fellowship".

These feelings are wrong and morbid. They ought not to be harboured at all but should be earnestly resisted There can be no doubt that they offer themselves as temptations. The only way to meet them is to say, "I am here, by the will of God" and to fix it in your heart that you can expect no blessing anywhere, but in the place that He appoints for you.

You are the *"prisoner for the Lord"* (Ephesians 4:1)[78] and so, when you pray for "all prisoners and captives" you will feel that you can pray for them since you have many needs and trials in common with them. As such, you are to *"walk worthy of the vocation wherewith ye are called, with all lowliness and meekness, with long-suffering, forbearing one another in love, endeavouring to keep the unity of the Spirit, in the bond of peace"* (Ephesians 4 :1).

"There is one body, and one Spirit, just as you are called in one hope of your calling, one Lord, one faith, one baptism, one God and Father of all, who is above all, and through all, and in you all" (Ephesians 4:1-6). While these verses tell you

---

[77]from The Creed

[78]Priscilla Maurice wrote the "prisoner of the Lord" as she was following King James Bible. More recent translations give the "prisoner for the Lord", which means something different.

your duties, they also at the same time, tell you how great your blessings are in the unity of the Church. They also tell you that sickness is not a state of isolation. For "*there is one body*" and the whole Church is one family, of which some are sick and some in health, each needing the other and unable to go on without the varied and reciprocal offices.

People often say that "you can just as well say your prayers at home". But it seems to you that this is just not true. Nevertheless, be assured that when God calls you to do so, "*He will make all grace abound towards you and will not suffer your soul to hunger*" (Deuteronomy 8:3). Jesus, who fed the five thousand with so few loaves and fishes will feed you. "*Bread shall be given you, and your water shall be sure*" (Isaiah 33:16 AV). God will feed you though often you may see no bread. However, this does not hinder you from receiving it. Sometimes, it may seem to you bitter bread, or very dry and it may seem rarely "*pleasant bread*" (Daniel 10:3 AV).

Fear not, though. The bread seems like this and "*though the scent of water*" (Job 14:9 AV) may be distant, yet He can feed you and give drink. He who gave you life will sustain it. He can exactly adapt the daily portion of bread to your need. He will make it sufficient to sustain you and to enable you to go on your way. Only do not seek to choose your food but let Him give you the "*the food that is needful for me*" (Proverbs 30:8).

You want to spend your Sundays differently from all other days but the difficulty is in how to do it. You have, perhaps, a great deal more quiet time and leisure for reading then, than on other days. But you cannot read all the time and you do not have enough variation in your daily life, for example in seeing friends, since you may scarcely even see your own family.

Have you ever considered then, as much as possible, making your Sunday as it would be if you could go to Church, and like your own past Sundays? You used to go to Church.

There was an appointed service, a guide and direction to your devotions and thoughts. A service that everyone joined in, not only in the particular church to which you went but throughout the world. Was it not intended for all the members of the Church? Then it belongs to you for you are a sick member of it.

If, when you know that the Service is beginning to be read at Church, you begin to read it too, then you can join with all those who are worshipping everywhere and you will cease to feel cut off and isolated. When you begin to do this, at first it can feel rather formal. It will possibly seem rather flat, without anyone to respond to, without hymns or music and you will take little, if any, pleasure in it.

Do not be disappointed and do not stop doing it because every time you try (after awhile) you will find more pleasure, profit and blessing in it and feel more as if you were joining "*the great congregation*" (Psalms 22:25 AV). Perhaps, too, you will find that reading a liturgy[79] and Scriptural readings slowly brings out new beauties which you never saw before. Your circumstances, too, may bring home to your heart some prayers and petitions which until now you had only "*heard with the hearing of the ear*" (Job 42:5 AV). During the liturgy, you can add the names of your own friends, separately naming them in your heart along with "the widows," the "fatherless children," the "sick," "all prisoners and captives". This will enhance it and enable you to be "*helpers of their joy*" (2 Corinthians 1:24 AV) and connect you with others who are *"sitting solitary"* (Lamentations 1:1).

Do not say to yourself that it would be too formal to read the Services in private when they are meant for public worship. Do not think that to use "forms" in private, and especially in a sick room, is a bondage to formality. If you are cut

---

[79]For example The Anglican *Book of Common Prayer*. We would suggest that you buy a small copy.

off from the Church by sickness then you have no part in her Services. It cannot be more formal to offer these prayers in private than in public, as they are for the whole Church, and therefore for you.

You may often complain that it is difficult to focus your thoughts and to offer up your own words in prayer. But in the formal Service are words designed for you. They are true and holy words which in all ages have been uttered, exactly suited to your desires, now and at all times. Sick people need guidance for their thoughts and words more than others do. They who have tried the plan of reading the Service during the hours of public worship, often speak about the exceeding blessing it has been to them.

If you are unable to read the whole Service, you can read some part of it. Perhaps you can read just the Confession and as much else as you have strength for. If you are able to read quite a lot at once, then, when you have read the Service, you can read a sermon. Then lie still for a time doing nothing. Then make sure that you take the refreshment of seeing someone in your family, or a friend who may come to visit you.

On Sunday afternoon or evening, you may be able to read the Service again and if you do, you will not find Sunday a tedious or a lonely day, but you will especially enjoy the rest and refreshment which this day offers and the relaxation from the work of other days.

To many sick people, the calm and rest of this holy day is peculiarly delightful. When they wake in the morning, they begin to feel the difference in it and to give thanks that on this day, the world may be shut out and other thoughts may fill up their hearts. They will be without interruption from outward things, or from daily domestic duties. They feel refreshed in spirit, and the better enabled to go on their way during the week to come, because of this *"day of refreshing from the presence of the Lord"* (Acts 3:19 AV).

The more you cultivate a love for Sunday, the more it will become a joyous day, a day of resources to be drawn upon all the week and rejoiced in when it returns. In this way, it will become the pledge and foretaste of the *"rest which remains"* (Hebrews 4:9), the rest which you long for. If at any time, you can get anyone to read the Service with you, it is a great help and pleasure. But you do not need this if you always consider yourself "in the congregation" and that you are truly one of the worshippers.

Always remember, too, that you are not alone, "All the company of Heaven laud and magnify His glorious name[80]". *"Therefore, since we are surrounded by so great a cloud of witnesses, let us also lay aside every weight, and sin which clings so closely, and let us run with endurance the race that is set before us, looking to Jesus, the founder and perfecter of our faith, who for the joy that was set before him endured the cross, despising the shame, and is seated at the right hand of the throne of God"* (Hebrews 12:1-2).

5.3 The Lord's Supper

When an illness first develops, those who have truly cared for the blessing of joining in the Communion, or Lord's Supper, at Church, keenly feel their absence from it. Especially when the days return for its accustomed celebration, they seem more than ever isolated and alone. This feeling may be, in part removed and much blessing rediscovered, by reading the Communion Service at the time when others are engaged in that service at the Church where you have been accustomed to worship. Or, if you do not have strength for the whole of it, at least read some portion of it.

You have been accustomed to think of this as merely a public service. But surely this cannot be the only view of it, since the Church has appointed a separate service (or at

---

[80]From the Book of Common Prayer

least an introductory service) for the Communion of the Sick, showing that it is for them too.

A rubric tells you that you may eat of The Lord's Supper by faith when you are truly stopped from doing it in reality. But sick people should not be content with merely receiving the elements. Those circumstances are rare and peculiar, in which it is not their bounden duty as well as their highest privilege and blessing, to eat the Body and to drink of the Blood of our Lord. Cases may occur where people are not visited by pastors or clergyman. Nevertheless, they are authorised by the Church to send for him and to ask him for this service. If circumstances make it impossible to get this blessing from the minister of the parish, at any rate, permission may be obtained to ask some friend, or someone through a friend, to minister the Communion Service, if not the elements to you.

There are very many obstacles and many great difficulties which almost every sick person finds in dealing with Communion. Generally speaking, most of them are either groundless, or may be overcome by prayer for guidance and strength. One hindrance is the peculiar shyness which sick people feel in mentioning their needs. This is probably is common to almost everyone ill and does not entirely depend on natural shyness. It arises from many causes.

The most frequent are: the dislike of giving trouble; the fear of seeming to make too much of yourself or your state; a dislike of speaking of 'self' and of your own wishes and a fear in case others should think that you are, or fancy yourself to be, more holy than you feel that you are. It may also arise from a feeling of awkwardness, from the thought that you cannot enjoy, or even take pleasure in, the Service unless it is in Church, a fear of interruptions and of not choosing a suitable time. There is the idea that you will wait until you are stronger or until perhaps you soon go to Church again. Lastly, there is the fear that by proposing such a Service, your friends should be alarmed and suppose that you think yourself to be dying.

One or more of these thoughts may have haunted the minds of most sick persons. A close examination of these difficulties would prove that some of them are quite groundless. It is like saying that a clergyman is not willing to do the work which his Master has given him to do, if we fear that he will count such service a burden.

If these fears were coming out of your own desires, you might fear the making too much of yourself, or your state. But remember who has commanded you: *"Do this in remembrance of Me"* (1 Corinthians 11:24 AV). Jesus said this in the upper chamber, on that last night when His sufferings had already begun. Do you think that He will count your obedience to His command self-indulgence? Remember what He wills and do not think just of how your fellow-creatures may judge you. But surely it is generally unreasonable to imagine such a thing of them? The dislike of speaking of yourself and about your own wishes, may go too far and become a morbid feeling which it certainly is, if it hinders us from doing the will of God.

Do not fear in case others think you more holy than you are, but try to be holy as He who is holy would have you be. Never mind the thoughts of your fellow creatures. *"I the Lord search the heart, I try the reins of the children of men"* (Jeremiah 17:10). Might there not also be in your feelings a mixture of fear, in case you should be expected to live more consistently and in a more holy way if you *"Proclaim His death"* (1 Corinthians 11:26) in this way?

Is this perhaps a device of the Adversary, who would hinder your growth? The feeling of awkwardness is very painful, but it soon wears off. The more frequent that Communion is administered, the less it is felt.

It is true, however, that it is far less like real Communion in a sick room, than in the Church. For the holy sanctuary, many coming together to the altar rail and all those associations are the greatest aid to worship. Nevertheless, when God calls anyone aside into their bedroom, He expects them to worship Him there, and not at Church. It is there that He meets with them, and blesses them.

They will not fail to find His presence, if they really expect it and believe in it. The fear of interruptions and of not choosing a suitable time, can be offset by setting apart a special time, which is the most free period of the day from interruptions and by making it a stated Service, at that time, more or less frequently according to circumstances.

Of course, in a short illness in which there is the hope of speedy recovery, it may be good to wait until you can go to Church. But in any long illness and especially in a life-long sickness, foregoing Communion is merely robbing yourself of a blessing which you never needed, perhaps so much, before.

As a guide, the Church of England specifies three times in the year as the least possible number for anyone to take Communion who considers himself as a member. Nor are the sick persons excluded from this order if they are members of the Church. It is easy to prevent causing alarm to your friends by the proposal if you first tell them that the desire is not from any idea of the immediate approach of death. You can tell them the desire comes from feeling that it is your highest duty and blessing.

It is a great mistake to wait until your dying hour before you avail yourself of so great a help in living to God and in suffering His holy will. Because Communion has so often been looked upon in this light, people are apt to fancy that it is required only in cases of dangerous sickness. There is no strength or help as great as Communion in a dying hour and it is a great blessing for those who have its comfort then. But we need grace and help and strength to suffer, as well as to die, for while living, we live unto the Lord.

Surely no slight hindrance, nothing that can possibly be overcome ought to prevent us from seeking this blessing and from fulfilling this command of our suffering and dying Lord and Master. What He has commanded He likewise desires. He says, *"I have earnestly desired to eat this Passover with you before I suffer"* (Luke 22:15). He is ready, He is inviting us and will be truly present with us.

He is ready. The unreadiness is only on our side. He is willing. The unwillingness is wholly on our part. He invites us and it is we who refuse.

The more frequently sick persons can take Communion, the more the feeling of strangeness and inability to enjoy the Service will decrease. They will eat and live. They will feel strengthened to carry on, on their weary way. They will be raised above suffering by *"looking to Jesus, the founder and perfecter of our faith, who for the joy that was set before him endured the cross, despising the shame, and is seated at the right hand of the throne of God"* (Hebrews 12:2).

In this way, they learn to *"endure as seeing Him who is invisible"* (Hebrews 11:27 AV) and to *"go from strength to strength, until they appear in Zion before God"* (Psalms 84:7 AV). Let no hindrances, no fears, no delays, rob you then of this your "bounden duty and service". Lay aside every weight and ask Him to overcome all difficulties for you. Look upon it as a duty and you will soon find that it can be fulfilled.

Beware of allowing yourself to make excuses, lest you should find that such excuses are not so easily accepted and allowed before God. If any special thing burdens your mind, any fear that some particular sin is a hindrance, the Church directs you to lay it before some discreet and learned minister of God's word.

Perhaps you have a fear lest your great bodily weakness should prevent you from attending and that you shall only give outward worship, your thoughts in the meantime either wandering, or being literally absent and beyond your control. Do not fear this. "*He knows your frame, and remembers that you are dust*" (Psalms 103:14 AV). He will only require and expect of you as much service and attention as you are able to give and He knows how much that is and expects no more. Sometimes sick people have found that they were raised far above their weakness and for the time being, enabled to forget it. It is a good plan to make it a special subject of prayer in advance, to ask that you may forget your body and yourself, that you may forget the presence of everyone and only be conscious of His presence, He who has invited you to meet Him and to "eat His flesh and drink His blood."

Even if it must be that you cannot attend to the whole Service, there will be a hallowed calm feeling shed around you and portions of it you will understand and enjoy. At times the blessing may be even greater afterwards than you were aware of at the time. Do not distress yourself when the Service is ended, or in time to come by thinking how little power of attention you had. Say rather like Peter, "*Lord, You know all things; you know that I love You*" (John 21:17). "Accept my poor, weak, broken service, not weighing my merits, but pardoning my offences, for the sake of Jesus Christ our Lord. Amen."

5.4 Prayer for Healing

People who are sick are often perplexed by the question of whether it is right to pray for healing. Some people urge the duty of doing so, as if they think they can "*take heaven by violence*" (Matthew 11:12 AV). Others, on the contrary, think that praying for healing is a proof of lack of submission to

God's will, of a belief that illness is sent by God and therefore we should not wish to get better.

Most certainly, if our Heavenly Father gave us everything that we ask just because we ask it, if He granted all our desires, just because He would not deny us anything, then we ought to ask for nothing but that which He has already given us and never tell Him our desires, in case when we think that we are asking for "a fish", it should prove "a stone".

Where then would be the comfort or the rest of prayer? But He gives us only those things that are really good for us, just as He withholds everything that would prove evil for us and He mercifully denies us when we pray for things which would not fulfil His gracious purposes towards us. So we need not fear to tell Him all our wishes, all our desires, and to leave it to Him to grant them, or to deny them as *"seems good in His sight"* (Luke 10:21 AV). We may *"rest in His love"* (Zephaniah 3:17) as much in sickness, as in all things.

It would show a lack of child-like confidence to keep back anything from God. So let us not fear to tell Him everything, to lay our wayward desires before Him and let Him teach us by His discipline whether these things seem good or not.

Therefore, if you desire to be healed, do not fear to tell Him so. If you share this with a friend, they may say, "This proves a sad lack of submission". But do not fear to tell God. Keep back nothing back from Him, as it is not sincere to do so. He requires truth *"in the inward being"* (Psalms 51:6). Ask Him, in this thing too, to conform you to His will, and then, surely, *"if in anything you think otherwise, God will reveal that also to you"* (Philippians 3:15).

When first a person is first 'visited' with sickness, it is a duty to pray that, if it be the will of God, he or she may be healed. Nor indeed only at the beginning of an illness. For the Church teaches us, even during the last period of an illness that we should pray, "We know, O Lord, that no work is impossible with you and that if you will it you can yet raise him or her up, and grant a longer continuance amongst us." So, in the Collect in the "Service for the Communion of the Sick" there is a prayer that "he may recover his bodily health". But added is "if it be Thy gracious will".

This seems a fit pattern for our prayers for healing. We ought to ask for it, since it would seem like an undervaluing of life if we did not. But we ought always to add "if it be Thy will" and to seek to be content in whatever form the answer comes. No fear of life and its cares and responsibilities, should keep us from this prayer and no imagination that the temptations of health are greater than those of sickness. We would indeed be novices in sickness to suppose this and not yet to have discovered that health is only a change of temptations and trials. No one can say which are the greatest temptations: those of health or those of sickness because they are so different that they cannot be compared. Besides, this would be underrating the power of God, who is able to strengthen us and to "keep us from falling" under any circumstances whatsoever. It is impossible, while life remains, ever to know that anyone will not recover or that their "sickness is unto death". But when it seems to be a case of life-long sickness, when we have once or twice asked that the 'thorn' of sickness may be removed and, if still, as in St. Paul's case, it is not permitted to *"depart from us"*, then let us be content with the assurance, *"My grace is sufficient for you"* (2 Corinthians 12:9).

Doubtless, after his prayers for physical healing, Paul was content and only asked, day by day, for the fulfilment of the promise and for ability to do and to suffer, his Master's will, in that state of life unto which it had pleased God to call him. The constant asking to have the thorn removed, either in his, or in our case might produce a very restless, dissatisfied spirit and a desire for that which it was not the will of God to give.

We must day by day, pray that God will give us the measure of grace and strength which we need to enable us to do His will.

Whenever you feel inclined to ask for healing, do not stop the desire or fear to share your wish with your heavenly Father. But leave it to Him to grant or to deny them, as He sees best for you.

Part VI - CONVALESCENCE

6.1 Its pleasures and Its trials

If you have ever experienced in the past, the trial of returning to health and life you may it find the thought difficult. For some people getting better from illness is a great trial[81].

You may, at some past period in your life, have had some serious illness which threatened your life. You may have been told that the illness was incurable and that recovery was impossible. You thought you had a few short hours which would be your last battle. It may be that you heard this prognosis with a very thankful heart. You did not fear death and had long waited the welcome summons to a better life.

Hour after hour passed away, but still you were still here on earth, to the surprise of your doctor and your friends. It seemed to them that you could not struggle through it. You thought that you were laying down your spiritual armour and that all temptations would soon be ended, all possibility of sinning would be left behind and that you should soon "*always be with the Lord*" (1 Thessalonians 4:17).

However, it pleased God to call you back to live longer. The crisis passed and you were told that you would now recover your bodily health. This was not easy. You had already taken leave of friends. You had finished so you thought, with earth and its allurements and now you must you return to it *"in the howling waste of the wilderness"* (Deuteronomy 32:10).

---

[81]It was considered acceptable in Victorian England to express a longing for death as a release from sin and as a reconciliation with chosen loved ones. Hence, longing for death, which might be considered a sign of depression and 'morbid' today, would have been reasonable in 1850.

Suddenly, you find it much harder to be content to live, than to be content and willing to die. "*My Father, if it be possible, let this cup pass from me; nevertheless, not as I will, but as you will*" (Matthew 26:39). "O take me where I would be; let me go to Thee; let me cease from sin; O let me be at rest forever[82]". Then the first severe inner conflict is over. You feel that God is Love and you can say, "*Thy will be done*".

Then comes the first glow of returning health. It brings feelings of joy and exhilaration, at least for a few hours or minutes of the day. But the exhaustion and consequent depression must be faced too. You feel the delight of the passing away of pain, of the return of independence and of the pleasure of doing something more for yourself each day. Above all, you have the congratulations and the great love and kindness of friends.

You never realised that they cared so much for you, that your life and your love were so important to them. You seem the one object of all your friends' attentions and you feel that the delight your recovery has given them and the new knowledge you have received of their love, was worth all the suffering. In other words, you have not obtained it at too great a price.

But the trial is not ended yet. These pleasant feelings, this first glow of returning health will pass away. In exchange, you will have exceeding weariness and languor which will induce great depression of spirits and a series of nervous and distressing feelings will arise out of your weakness. This again will lie heavy on your mind. Instead of the pleasure of finding that each day you can do more and more, for some time it will seem to you either that you can do less each day, or that you are neither getting better or worse.

You will seem to grow weaker in mind and body. You imagine that friends are less loving and considerate than they were at first. You forget though, that at first, in the time of

---

[82] We cannot yet identify where this quotation is taken from.

Sickness: its Trials and Blessings

anxiety, they thought that they should only have you for a few more days and their usual agendas were laid aside and their thoughts centred in you.

It cannot continue like this. You must now be content to have that care scattered through your life, which was gathered up into a short space and to receive, almost unconsciously, the gentle shower of love from hour to hour, instead of the full tide which flowed so delightfully upon you.

As for you, you must return to the bustle and fluster of life again and all its temptations which used to assault you will return now. You will have the trial of finding that you are just as open to temptations as before, with, it seems to you, less strength to meet them.

You thought that in sickness you had lost your susceptibility to temptations. They did not assail you so much and you did not perceive that the reason for this was that you had a change of temptations, a change of trials, but not an exemption from them. You thought that you were much more changed and renewed by illness than it now appears to you to be the case. When you were very ill, spiritual realities were ever present and the unseen world seemed very close. Friends at rest seemed around your bed. Sometimes they alone seemed real to you and you had far closer communion with them than with those about you.

You thought that this state was so much a part of you, that it would always last and that the power of the world over you was gone and all its charm broken, never to be renewed. But now, the spiritual realities dwindle and seem to fade daily more and more from your sight.

The world slowly and imperceptibly gains its hold of you, and earthly desires fasten upon you. The cares and business of the earth engross you and your lawful calling is fast filling up your heart and because it is your lawful calling, it is the more insinuating and dangerous.

You have not yet recovered your full strength. Every little demand weighs heavily on you. Each little fatigue is very great and you become irritable and fretful, dissatisfied with yourself, and everyone around.

Then you look back at the time lately, in which you seemed so different. You think yourself in a far worse state than you were before and you are deeply discouraged. You think that friends misunderstand you and you say, *"I loathe my life"* (Job 10:1). You thought that you had entered the "river" of passing over, that the soles of your feet were wet, that you had gone deeper down and yet, after all that you were called back to life. You have been called back for you know not how long. All that seemed done and finished must now begin again.

You say to yourself that you shall never believe it again when you are told that you are dying, and that until 'the last enemy' has actually done its work, you shall be always expecting that another 'disappointment'.

It is better to realize that the times and the seasons are hidden from you. Only do not let this understanding make you unwatchful. Let it lead you to much more earnest watching because *"concerning that day or that hour, no one knows, not even the angels in heaven, nor the Son, but only the Father"* (Mark 13:32).

Much of your sense of discouragement is physical and arises from the return to duties, fatigues and enduring the wear and tear of life with a weakened body and shattered nerves. Have patience with this state as it will pass away gradually as strength returns. Impatience added to it will greatly add to your trial and distress. It must happen.

Take it as a necessary humiliation, as a proof that there is much still to be corrected in you, before you are ready for the Master's presence. Lie down in quiet submission to His Fatherly correction as He will teach you very much by this process if you will only *"Take my yoke upon you, and learn from me, for I am gentle and lowly in heart, and you will find rest for your souls"* (Mark 11:29).

You still need to be shown what was in your heart and you must learn it in His way not in your own. Believe also, that by all this discipline, He is preparing you for life, for serving Him better and for understanding and helping your fellows in faith more than you have done so far.

God has work yet for you to do, so do it cheerfully and without complaining. Be very thankful to be employed for Him, in any way that He pleases.

6.2 Being Called Back to Life - how to Accept Life Again

There are some who have desired to die for many years, who have been brought very close to death and yet have been called back to life and learned to love it. Their struggle has been a very difficult one.

At first, when they were called back, they could scarcely bear the trial and its extreme disappointment. They had fully thought to go to "a better place" and now, for a while, they must stay. They thought that their pain and suffering was nearly over. Now there is the prospect of its long continuance. They had thought that they should soon be out of the reach of temptation, but they are called to return to them all. One step more and they believed that their weary, earthly pilgrimage would be at an end. Instead, it stretches before them like a sea without a shore.

It may be that they have had the expectation of immediate departure. Instead, they are called by God to lie seemingly in the arms of death for weeks or months, all the time, eagerly looking for the welcome summons and growing impatient of the long delay.

They may, perhaps, have had very good reasons and desires. They may really have desired to *"depart and be with Christ"*

(Philippians 1:23 AV) and not from lower motives. But even in such a desire, there may be an unchastened eagerness, a lack of entire submission which the Refiner saw necessary to purge out and purify. He accepts, most lovingly, the desire to be with Him, though He may not see fit to grant it right now. Instead He makes His child wait a little longer, until their will is wholly one with His and with what He wishes. That and that alone they will wish also.

It is only for our blessing that He keeps us here on earth, for the Lord has said, *"Father, I desire that they also, whom you have given me, may be with me where I am, to see my glory that you have given me because you loved me before the foundation of the world"* (John 17:24). Jesus' will is to have all His children gathered into His presence. However, His love often waits long for the fulfilment, so that they may be perfected. It is often a long time before the soul perceives this truth. In the meantime, the soul may be tormented by hard thoughts about God, by impatience at the delay, by restlessness, discontent, weariness of life, disappointment, and, at times, rebellion against His holy will.

But He will not leave us in this state. He will *"subdue our iniquities"* (Micah 7:19 AV) and bring our wills to *"the obedience of faith"* (Romans 16:26).

The Almighty God, who alone can order the unruly wills and affections of sinful men will order ours. With some, it is a very long process, with others much more rapid. But that *"patient waiting for Christ"* (2 Thessalonians 3:5 AV) the Lord alone can "direct the heart to." It is not soon attained. The steps are often very slow and the disappointments very great. It often seems like walking in very wet weather among puddles: we seem to go back as many steps as we go forward.

First, there may be an occasional willingness to live, which alternates with a real desire to die. Then, gradually the willingness may be more persistent until it is understood that

Sickness: its Trials and Blessings

God is speaking, saying, "To remain in the flesh is more necessary on your account". Then the soul answers, *"Convinced of this, I know that I will remain and continue with you all, for your progress and joy in the faith"* (Philippians 1:24,25). It is this assurance of the will of God that changes our mind. It does not transform the character less than the mind. Instead, it produces a quiet submission and chastens the whole person. There is no longer a struggle, no longer the sense of "This is His will, but that is mine; I must submit, for I cannot help it. O that He would will it otherwise!".

This rebellious thought becomes "This is His will and because it is His will, therefore it is my will. My will leads me astray, so I give it up forever, and seek to know only His will. I always find rest in His Will as everything else is unrest to me. I can rest in His love, and wait until He calls me".

Besides the certainty of it being His will, there comes a deep sense of thankfulness at being allowed to do anything for Him, to serve Him in any way, whether through suffering, or in whatever form service may come. To work for God is good and pleasant and seems a thing to be thankful for, a great honour.

The work may be hidden, but day by day, hour by hour, it will be revealed. The work and the strength will be apportioned equally and sent together. Then, also, there is a deep sense of having been most unfit to depart at the time when it was eagerly desired. A feeling of shame and wonder, too, that you could ever have thought yourself ready to go, when now, in looking back, you see how your will was at variance with the will of God, how much you were actually seeking self, ease and rest, when you thought that you were seeking God.

How full of self-delusion the past seems! At times you can scarcely think about it, to remember how much better you thought yourself and your state than you had justification for and how you imagined it was "well" with your soul, when you now see that it was far from well.

You feel very thankful that you were not cut off then, before you knew more of God and of yourself, before your will was conformed to His will. You feel now that you know nothing, that you have no idea what is the best for you, that you would not choose if you could but prefer to leave yourself in His hands, either to serve Him, by suffering so long as He sees fit, or to return to active service in the world. In this state of mind, you leave the time of your departure wholly to Him, engage in no speculations about it, but grow, day by day, in love towards Him, so that for your love to Him the time shall seem to you only one day.

Now you do not want to die. You only want to have no separate will and to lose yourself in God. Formerly you looked on your sojourn here as "absence from God", almost entire separation. You felt that you were always preparing to be with Him, but were yet far off from Him and this added greatly to the weariness of life and the eagerness for death.

Now you have learned that He is always present with you, though you do not always realise it and that the one object of your life should be to live with Him now, to feel that He is "*about your path and your lying down, and acquainted with all your ways*" (Psalm 139:3 AV). You feel that you never need be alone and can say, "*I am not alone, for the Father is with me*" (John 8:16 AV).

You have learnt, to some extent, to understand His nearness to you, His tender sympathy, His sharing all your thoughts and your very heart and that in Him all your deepest cravings are satisfied. You will not lead a sad and solitary life because He will always be with you, your "Friend "and "Counsellor, "your Lord and Master" and even your "Husband."

You have learnt that the more you learn of Him here, the more ready you will be to enter into and enjoy His presence in Heaven. There is so much to learn about Him and about you, here. You would be frightened in case you do not learn everything and should die too soon. If you did not know the great patience of your Teacher, that His Love is so wonderful, that He will have you *"conformed to His image"* (Romans 8:29 AV).

At times, you are worried that there is something wrong in this change of heart about dying. You are concerned in case it proves a decrease of your love for Him and proves that you desire less to be with Him. But it is not the case. You have the deepest reason to give thanks that you have been brought into this condition of heart, though you may have passed through fearful conflicts to attain it.

Remember, too, that however firm this state of mind may seem, it is subject to fluctuation and that sudden temptations to impatience and self-pity may seize you and take hold of you by coming upon you without warning. There is no state, this side of the grave, in which we can cease to stand in our "watch tower." *"Watch and pray that you may not enter into temptation. The spirit indeed is willing, but the flesh is weak"* (Mark 14:38). *"As for you, always be sober-minded, endure suffering"* (2 Timothy 4:5). "Work your work betimes, and in His time He will give you your reward" (Ecclesiastes 2:30).

You will find work to do if you will constantly look to God to give you your hourly portion of it, to show you what He would have you to do. If you are constantly looking out for it, it will come to you, in bearing suffering and in self-control, in little acts of self-denial, in helping others and in ways for which you will get no credit. For theirs will be the work that is seen and yours the work that is unseen. This is work done in the continual renunciation of your own will and through living for others, instead of for yourself.

All that you have learned in your most acute sickness, all that you are learning now, in its lengthened effects of debilitating weakness which disables you from the delights of active Christian ministry, will help you in what now lies before you.

Part VII - DEATH

7.1 The fear of death - the fear of it taken away

There are some Christian believers who have never known what it is to fear death. They have seemed to be very near to dying, but have always rejoiced. They have hailed the Angel of Death as a bright presence, spoken of death as a joyful prospect, of death itself as "beautiful". They have never had any sympathy with those who have spoken fearfully of it. They have thought such feelings either lack of moral courage, lack of faith or a proof of earthliness of heart. They may have made hard judgements of those who did fear death. They say that they cannot understand how anyone can fear death. But their turn comes, *"Fear and trembling come upon me, and horror overwhelms me"* (Psalms 55:5). *"My heart is struck down like grass and has withered; I forget to eat my bread"* (Psalms 102:4). Now their judgements come back.

Perhaps, there may be no particular cause for you at present, for this "sudden fear." You may not be more ill than you have been, nothing may have occurred to stimulate such thoughts. But you find suddenly that its fear has seized upon your soul and there is no escape from it. Death has fastened his eye upon you and there is no escaping the fixedness of his searching look. You must meet it and for the first time it makes you quail.

You may have met it before, so why then should you fear to meet it now? You don't know. This time, death comes to you as a perfectly new apparition. It is the exceeding and indescribable vagueness of it that terrifies you. You feel that something is going to grasp you but what, is unknown. No one can tell you much about it because no one has returned to tell what they passed through at death. You seem to be all alone and you tremble at this exceeding loneliness. *"A hor-*

rible dread" (Psalms 55:5 AV) comes upon you; your whole nature, both in body and in soul, trembles to its very centre.

There is the awareness of personal sinfulness, the sense of unfitness to meet God, the unpreparedness to die, the multitude of personal faults, the evil temper, the bad thoughts and habits. There are the recollection of innumerable sins, of great omissions and lukewarmness in religious duties, the scant love and gratitude given to God and the imperfection of repentance. All these make us tremble at the thought of going to give our account to God. We feel as if it were impossible that we could be saved.

When we come, as it were, into the presence of death, our whole consciousness is penetrated with a sense of sin. We see not only the evil we have done but the good we have left undone. The good that we have tried to do, we see for the first time, revealed by some strange and searching light, in which it all looks blemished, marred and sullied. Well, let this sin simply drive you closer to His Cross. Give up yourself, your sin and your will into His hands.

He will not leave you to yourself, He will not forsake you. He is near and that justifies you. *"And the daughter of Zion is left like a booth in a vineyard, like a lodge in a cucumber field, like a besieged city. If the Lord of hosts had not left us a few survivors, we should have been like Sodom, and become like Gomorrah"* (Isaiah 1:8,9).

Let us ask ourselves, *"Who, then, shall separate me from the love of God in Jesus Christ?"* (Romans 8:39). There is nothing that is able to. Though all powers of hell be against me for my unutterable guilt, all His holy powers are on my side. God the Father loves me and gave His Son for me. God the Son loves me and gave Himself for me. God the Holy Spirit loves me and has regenerated, prevented, restrained, converted me. The ever-blessed Trinity loves me and desires my salvation. All heavenly powers and all holy angels love and rejoice over one penitent soul.

Sickness: its Trials and Blessings

The whole world unseen is benign and blessed, full of love to sinners, *'of whom I am chief'* *(1 Timothy 1:15)*[83]. So I give myself into the hands of a boundless love. As an infinite misery, I cast myself upon an infinite mercy. This is my comfort and it is all sufficing.

So though some may desire death, others recoil from it in their inmost souls. They may desire life in any form of suffering, rather than meet death. In some people, there is an instinctive, a natural fear of death due to which they are *"subject to lifelong slavery"* (Hebrews 2:15). The very idea of death is a terror to them and they can scarcely bear to hear "death" mentioned. They have tried by faith and earnest prayers to overcome this dread, but all their life it remains with them until they are brought into the very presence of death.

Then generally, either the fear is removed or the soul that has been ever dreading the last hour, passes out of life unknowingly and without any suffering of body or mind. There may be instances to the contrary but they are rare. All their prayers offered day by day, that the fear of death might be removed are answered at the last. Their prayers were not in vain. They were heard and were not forgotten by God.

Many people have a peculiar dread of a last illness. They know that it must come, but their soul recoils from it. They would like to die suddenly, to escape it. Does the fear of pain that makes them afraid? The thought that, then, when the last hour is drawing near, pain will put forth its full strength, a strength that they have never known before. Does your whole soul recoil from this thought? He who said, *"My Father, if it be possible, let this cup pass from me; never-*

---

[83]The English Standard Version translates St Paul's words as: *"The saying is trustworthy and deserving of full acceptance, that Christ Jesus came into the world to save sinners, of whom I am the foremost"*.

theless, not as I will, but as you will" (Matthew 26:39) knows and understands your fear.

He tasted this fear of death that He might understand it, so that not one of His children might ever pass through this fear, alone. Is it the helplessness of those last hours? The unspeakable suffering which no heart but your own can share, which distresses you? The possibility of doing or saying something wrong at the end that haunts you? Of being unable, through broken speech, to convey your meaning?

Fear not: there is One who knows and understands it all, who looks at your thoughts and intentions and looks into your heart the most tenderly when He knows that no one else can. You have given yourself to Him. Fear not. Jesus will not leave you at the last hour for He has called you to it and He will lead you through. He said, *"I have a baptism to be baptised with, and how great is my distress until it is accomplished"* (Luke 12:50). It was accomplished in Him.

When He said, *"It is finished"* (John 19:30 AV) then the loneliness of the deepest darkness of death was finished for each of His followers. He will come to fetch you, so trust yourself to Him. He says, *"I am with you always, to the end of the age"* (Matthew 28:20) *"Let not your hearts be troubled. Believe in God; believe also in me"* (John 14:1).

It is pointless to think about what you would prefer. God will choose for you and be sure that He will choose the very best thing which you will afterwards see was the best. Do not judge your spiritual state by your desire for death, or for life. This leads to false opinions.

For those to whom life has been very sweet, who have enjoyed it, who have had many ties, especially the nearest and closest ties, such as husband, wife or children; for those who see a fair and bright prospects ahead of them and have comforts and earthly blessings around them, it is a difficult thing to give up life with a willing and glad heart, or even, with the whole soul, and say, "Thy will be done".

While for others, whose ties have been few, whose earthly prospects have been darkened, who have no one depending on them and no one who loves them best, it may be very easy to be willing and even a "release" to lay aside their weary, worn-out body.

No one ought on the one hand to say that it is sinful not to be more desirous to depart or on the other, that it is a proof of readiness and submission to wish to depart. You sometimes, perhaps, say to your friends, "Do not pray for me to live." Ought you to have such a choice?

Is it not better to ask God to give us either life or death, sickness or health, as it pleases Him? It has been thought these words are a proof of a desire for, and readiness to depart, but surely it is a higher state to leave everything to Him and to know nothing yourself, what you would prefer. We are poor judges. Let us not judge and leave it to Him who has *"appointed a set time"* (Job 14:13 AV) for us and will "remember" us.

As for ourselves, let the true language of our hearts be -

> *"Let me never choose, either to live or die.*
>
> *Bind or bruise, in Thy hands I lie.*
>
> *For my blinded choice, like myself, would be.*
>
> *I rejoice that Thou choose for me"*[84].

7.2 A public death-bed, and the desire to choose its circumstances

It is not only death that some people fear, but there is a peculiar dread from a death-bed surrounded by many people.

---

[84]We cannot identify the source of these lines. It is not impossible that Priscilla Maurice wrote them.

How often they think, "If I can only die in the night, or if there were such and such a person with me, or only one friend and a pastor to commend my soul to God, then death would seem much easier. But I dread the effect that the presence of many people might have on me, their weeping and sorrow will fill my thoughts and oppress and sadden my mind. I feel as if I could not bear it. Then, too, I fear that I will be tempted to say things merely to give them pleasure, or for my words to be remembered and I fear that they would be empty words. I am fearful too, in case in my last hour I should dishonour my Lord and Master, *"the God who has been my shepherd all my life long to this day"* (Genesis 48:15). I am frightened too that in my last hours there should be an element of impatience, or evil words, even in a delirium when those fearful pains come which will separate the soul from the body".

These are quite natural fears and are not inconsistent with true faith. These fears are not peculiar to you. From the intuitive knowledge of the wants of all her children, the Church teaches us to pray "You know, O Lord, the secrets of our hearts; shut not Thy merciful ears to our prayer; but spare us Lord most holy, O God most mighty, O holy and merciful Saviour, Thou most worthy Judge eternal, suffer us not, at our last hour, for any pains of death to fall from Thee". We can offer this prayer up continually now and can be sure that it will be answered, when the time of need actually arrives.

Beware of the temptation to want to choose the circumstances of your death. You cannot choose them, even if you could. At the time of death, you will be just where your heavenly Father sees fit. He will call you either by night or by day, alone or in company, sleeping or waking, as *"seems good in His sight"* (Luke 10:21 AV). Leave it all to Him.

Do not morbidly try to imagine the possible circumstances, or the pains or the words. Do not judge from your present symptoms what turn they must take or what suffering they must bring. All things may be wholly different. Another illness may be the appointed "messenger" to call you away to Him. You may be in a place where you have never yet been, with people you have never yet seen. It is useless to speculate about it or to distress your mind with forms of trial which may never come upon you. Of only this be sure: that you will not be alone for *"The Father will be with you"* (John 16:32).

7.3 The Right Way of Viewing Death

It is most awesome to meet death because death is the *"wages of sin"* (Romans 6:23 AV) and to meet that last full judgement with nothing to offer in return, except the very thing which has brought the punishment, sin itself. By one man sin entered into the world and death entered the world through sin. So death *"passed upon all men"* (Romans 5:12 AV).

But is there no other way of looking on death? Yes, there is; *"thanks be to God, who gives us the victory through our Lord Jesus Christ"* (1 Corinthians15:57). He has overcome the sharpness of death and opened the kingdom of Heaven to all believers. And He, who is our Judge, is also our Saviour. *"She will bear a son, and you shall call his name Jesus, for he will save his people from their sins"* (Matthew1:21). He has said, *"Shall I ransom them from the power of Sheol? Shall I redeem them from Death? O Death, where are your plagues? O Sheol, where is your sting? Compassion is hidden from my eyes"* (Hosea 13:14) *"O death, where is your victory? O death, where is your sting?"* (1 Corinthians 15:55). *"Fear not, for I am with you; be not dismayed, for I am your God; I will strengthen you, I will help you, I will uphold you with my righteous right hand"* (Isaiah 41:10).

He has passed through death. "*He tasted death for every man*" (Hebrews 2:2 AV). He has redeemed it from its loneliness so that from henceforth, no one can go down into death alone; for *"even there your hand shall lead me, and your right hand shall hold me"* (Psalms 139;10). *"He is near that justifies thee"* (Isaiah 50:8 AV).

Jesus is the companion of everyone whom He calls into the dark valley. *"Even though I walk through the valley of the shadow of death, I will fear no evil, for you are with me; your rod and your staff, they comfort me"* (Psalms 23:4). All the weariness and languor of dying, all its unutterable pains, all its exceeding vagueness, all its fears and temptations, all its darkness and dreariness, He passed through, Himself. He knows every step of the way and He comes to fetch each one Himself. He *"when he has found it, he lays it on his shoulders, rejoicing"* (Luke 15:5). It is a *"wilderness, a land of deserts and pits, a land of drought and deep darkness, a land that no one passes through, where no man dwells"* (Jeremiah 2:6), a path in which no one can truly help another. Yet He who has gone every step of the way knows the way Himself and He will conduct each of His children safely through it.

Do not fear not to go down with Him into the dark river. It may prove rough for a season, the waves may threaten to drown you. But fear not. He is with you. *"Fear not, I am the one who helps you"* (Isaiah 41:13).

Whatever weakness you may be called to pass through, He will be the *"strength of your heart"* (Psalms 73:26 AV) He will sustain you however your body may fail. In deepest weakness you will meet strength such as you never knew before, for the Almighty Lord will be with you and strengthen you. You will never know the fullness of His strength until you know your utmost weakness. Then His *"strength be made perfect in your weakness"* (2 Corinthians 12:9 AV).

The way is short, shorter than you can imagine, until you reach the end. You will surely find that a *"highway shall be there"* (Isaiah 35:8 AV) for He with whom and in whom you walk, is "The Way." Walk in that way and in a little time you shall *"return and come to Zion with singing; everlasting joy shall be upon your head; you shall obtain gladness and joy, and sorrow and sighing shall flee away"* (Isaiah 35:10). You shall be "delivered from the burden of the flesh" and be in "joy and felicity" forever. *"He will wipe away every tear from their eyes, and death shall be no more, neither shall there be mourning, nor crying, nor pain any more, for the former things have passed away"* (Revelation 21:4).

Sickness: its Trials and Blessings

APPENDIX

Suggestions to those ministering to the sick and dying

It is generally thought that in states of exhaustion, the mind is in the same exhausted a state as the body. But this is by any means always the case. There may be such entire loss of bodily power, that the sick person may be unable to move hand or foot, or make any movement of the lips or any sign at all. Even doctors with their more exact means of judging can think a patient is entirely unconsciousness. In fainting or in epileptic fits, this is usually the case, but it is not the case in the long and weary attacks of exhaustion to which some patients are subject.

At times, when life seems to be ebbing fast, the mind is often undisturbed. It is able to have closer contact with the unseen world, than when the eyes are open to the visible world. This may not be through any act of prayer, but through a perfect sense of the presence of God, of resting in His Love. It may be a consciousness of death being near, of the unseen world close at hand, of life passing away and of yielding up the body, soul and spirit into the hands of "*the faithful Creator*" (1 Peter 4:19).

All this and much more may, be passing between the soul and God, while friends at the side of the bed think that the mind is inactive. This being the case, it is of great importance that nurses and visitors should recognise this and learn how to treat the patient. Here are some suggestions:

> a) you should say nothing in the room which they would not wish the sick person to hear or would not say to them, at another time. For it is certain that in all states, excepting in cases of deafness, hearing is the sense that goes last and the first that returns;

b) you should avoid needlessly disturbing or troubling the patient. Very little can be done. Gently applying restoratives to the forehead, put hot bottles near the feet, rub the hands and feet if they are numb or cold, but avoiding this, when they are not. Avoid touching the person as it often causes distress and a great sense of additional fatigue. Besides this, nothing can be done. Nothing remains but quietness, waiting with patience, and occasionally attempting to serve, in these ways.

d) Much may be done for the comfort and soothing of a person in this state, by someone beside them either occasionally reading a prayer of intercession, or a verse of Holy Scripture or repeating a few words. But this must be done very slowly, distinctly and with intervals. It should not be done in a whisper or in a loud voice, but clearly and calmly, and the sentences should be kept very short. No one can explain the comfort of this, without having had it tried in their own case.

e) Questions should only rarely be asked and as soon as it is seen that they cannot be answered, those in attendance should say: "Do not try to answer, as I see you cannot". Otherwise, a sense is left in the mind of those in this state that something undone which ought to be attempted, and the impossibility of it becomes painful.

f) When a question is asked, it should not be done suddenly, but the hand gently touched or taken hold of whilst speaking.

g) When a person is recovering, it should not be attempted to make them speak too soon. A few gentle words, perhaps of thankfulness for their being better should be said, but no effort should be expected and

> the utmost quietness observed for a long time afterwards.
>
> h) Except the last sentence, all that has been said applies equally in the case of most of the dying.

Often weakness and exhaustion is so great that there is scarcely a sign of life. Friends are eager to hear some "last words", and, if not that at least to receive some sign of faith or hope, or love. Perhaps some question is asked as to the hope that is in them and it is said, "If you cannot answer, press my hand." Perhaps, the effort is made, the request is fulfilled. It may have cost a very great effort to a dying person. It may have distracted their thoughts very painfully to make this effort and may have withdrawn them, in part, from communion with God and with the unseen world. And why was this asked? Because we are apt to *"seek after a sign"* (Mark 8:12 AV).

Someone's life is the true evidence of their salvation and not their inner state when the soul is passing out of consciousness.

The holiest souls may have a last conflict with sin. They may be spoken to by God about sin, at that moment. They may utter words which will give no comfort to their friends. So leave them to God to teach them and leave it to Him to give them the words to speak, if in these, they glorify His Name. If they can speak, they will. If not, give their silence to Him in faith, for He can interpret it.

If the dying cannot have the help and comfort of the presence and service of a minister or pastor, you may help them greatly by speaking to them words of prayer or reading a Holy Scripture, not chiefly soothing words or words of mere comfort.

Speak to them of sin, of pardon, of *"the blood of Christ which cleanses from all sin"* (1 John 1:7) of the name of Jesus, of the love of Christ for sinners, of Him who has overcome the sharpness of death, and opened the kingdom of heaven to all believers, "*of His victory over sin*" of *"death having no more dominion over them"* (Romans 6:9 AV).

If a dying person can speak and speak to you, he or she will. If not, trust them to God and it shall be well with them and with you also. Remember, that the answer has been given to the question, *"When shall I come to appear before the presence of God?"* (Psalms 42:2 AV) and it is, *"Behold, I stand at the door and knock"* (Revelations 3:20).

This time is a moment full of awe. Therefore be careful not to come between the soul and God, or to hinder someone from hearing His voice. God has taken the soul aside. He is speaking. Therefore *"Let your words be few"* (Ecclesiastes 5:2). If any sounds can reach their ear, now, if any words can touch their heart, they will be His words, and not yours. Speak only in His words, and not in your own. The soul is about to be left alone with God, so let it draw near to Him and to commit itself to Him and to lie down in His arms in peace.

You may say, "We can learn so much from the words of the dying since death-beds are so edifying". Yes, they are if God speaks through the dying, but not otherwise. Do not doubt, but earnestly believe, that, if God has words for the dying to say, He will give them the power to say them and the words will come with power into your heart.

But leave it all to Him. Do not interfere with His work. try not to put too much dependence on last words. They may be only the dying words of mortal agony. They may be groans which can, or which cannot be uttered. It is not in this way that you are to look for a "blessing" from death-beds.

Look at death as the "*wages of sin*" (Romans 6:23) as a bitter and awful sentence which has been passed upon all Mankind. Then look at it as that which Christ came to conquer so that we may say: *"Thanks be to God who gives us the vic-*

tory, through Jesus Christ our Lord" (1 Corinthians 15:57 AV).

Look at death as that to which you will come yourself, that for which you must prepare. Look at it as a time of near and solemn communion with God when you are called to go down, into the valley of the shadow of death.

At that river, you must part company and leave the soul of your brother or sister in the hands of Jesus who has *"tasted death for everyone"* (Hebrews 2:9) and who will carry each soul safely into His own kingdom. Look at death as bringing you very near to the unseen world, as if opening a door to Heaven for you, and it will be your fault if it is ever again closed.

Look at death as teaching you the meaning of the words: *"I believe in the Holy Catholic Church, the communion of saints, the forgiveness of sins, the resurrection of the body, and the life everlasting*[85]*"*.

THE END

---

[85]from The Creed

Sickness: its Trials and Blessings

Sickness: its Trials and Blessings

THE ORDER FOR THE VISITATION OF THE SICK

> *Priscilla Maurice based many of her teachings and observations on this Service. This version is taken from 1662 Book of Common Prayer and is not modernised so that the seriousness of the original language should speak for itself.*

When any person is sick, notice shall be given thereof to the Minister of the Parish who, coming into the sick person's house, shall say,

Peace be to this house, and to all that dwell in it.

When he cometh into the sick person's presence he shall say, kneeling down,

Remember not, Lord, our iniquities, nor the iniquities of our forefathers. Spare us, good Lord, spare thy people, whom thou hast redeemed with thy most precious blood, and be not angry with us for ever.

> Answer. Spare us, good Lord.

Then the Minister shall say,

Let us pray. Lord, have mercy upon us. Christ, have mercy upon us. Lord, have mercy upon us.

Our Father, which art in heaven, Hallowed be thy Name. Thy kingdom come. Thy will be done in earth, as it is in heaven. Give us this day our daily bread. And forgive us our trespasses, As we forgive them that trespass against us. And lead us not into temptation; But deliver us from evil. Amen.

> Minister. O Lord, save thy servant
>
> Answer. Which putteth his trust in thee.
>
> Minister. Send him help from thy holy place
>
> Answer. And evermore mightily defend him.
>
> Minister. Let the enemy have no advantage of him;

Sickness: its Trials and Blessings

Answer. Nor the wicked approach to hurt him.

Minister. Be unto him, O Lord, a strong tower.

Answer. From the face of his enemy.

Minister. O Lord, hear our prayers.

Answer. And let our cry come unto thee.

Minister. - O Lord, look down from heaven, behold, visit, and relieve this, thy servant. Look upon him with the eyes of thy mercy, give him comfort and sure confidence in thee, defend him from the danger of the enemy, and keep him in perpetual peace and safety; through Jesus Christ our Lord. Amen.

Hear us, Almighty and most merciful God and Saviour; extend thy accustomed goodness to this thy servant who is grieved with sickness. Sanctify, we beseech thee, this thy fatherly correction to him; that the sense of his weakness may add strength to his faith, and seriousness to his repentance. That, if it shall be thy good pleasure to restore him to his former health, he may lead the residue of his life in thy fear and to thy glory: or else, give him grace so to take thy visitation, that, after this painful life ended, he may dwell with thee in life everlasting; through Jesus Christ our Lord. Amen.

Then shall the Minister exhort the sick person after this form, or other like.

Dearly beloved, know this, that Almighty God is the Lord of life and death, and of all things to them pertaining, as youth, strength, health, age, weakness, and sickness. Wherefore, whatsoever your sickness is, know you certainly, that it is God's visitation. And for what cause soever this sickness is sent unto you; whether it be to try your patience for the example of others, and that your faith may be found in the day of the Lord laudable, glorious, and honourable, to the increase of glory and endless felicity; or else it be sent unto

Sickness: its Trials and Blessings

you to correct and amend in you whatsoever doth offend the eyes of your heavenly Father; know you certainly, that if you truly repent you of your sins, and bear your sickness patiently, trusting in God's mercy, for his dear Son Jesus Christ's sake, and render unto him humble thanks for his fatherly visitation, submitting yourself wholly unto his will, it shall turn to your profit, and help you forward in the right way that leadeth unto everlasting life.

If the person visited be very sick, then the Curate may end his exhortation in this place, or else proceed.

Take therefore in good part the chastisement of the Lord: For (as Saint Paul saith in the twelfth Chapter to the Hebrews) whom the Lord loveth he chasteneth, and scourgeth every son whom he receiveth. If ye endure chastening, God dealeth with you as with sons; for what son is he whom the father chasteneth not? But if ye be without chastisement, whereof all are partakers, then are ye bastards, and not sons. Furthermore, we have had fathers of our flesh, which corrected us, and we gave them reverence: shall we not much rather be in subjection unto the Father of spirits, and live? For they verily for a few days chastened us after their own pleasure; but he for our profit, that we might be partakers of his holiness. These words, good brother, are written in holy Scripture for our comfort and instruction; that we should patiently, and with thanksgiving, bear our heavenly Father's correction, when soever by any manner of adversity it shall please his gracious goodness to visit us. And there should be no greater comfort to Christian persons, than to be made like unto Christ, by suffering patiently adversities, troubles, and sicknesses. For he himself went not up to joy, but first he suffered pain; he entered not into his glory before he was crucified. So truly our way to eternal joy is to suffer here with Christ; and our door to enter into eternal life is gladly to die with Christ; that we may rise again from death, and dwell with him in everlasting life. Now therefore, taking your sickness, which is thus profitable for you, patiently, I exhort you, in the Name of God, to remember the profession which you made unto God in your Baptism. And forasmuch as after this life there is an account to be given unto the righteous judge, by whom all must be judged, without respect of persons, I require you to examine yourself and your estate, both toward God and man; so that, accusing and condemning yourself for your own faults, you may find mercy at our heavenly Father's hand for Christ's sake, and not be accused and condemned in that fearful judgement. Therefore I shall rehearse to you the Articles of our Faith, that you may know whether you do believe as a Christian man should, or no.

Here the Minister shall rehearse the Articles of the Faith, saying thus,

Dost thou believe in God the Father Almighty, Maker of heaven and earth? And in Jesus Christ his only-begotten Son our Lord? And that he was conceived by the Holy Ghost, born of the Virgin Mary; that he suffered under Pontius Pilate, was crucified, dead, and buried; that he went down into hell, and also did rise again the third day; that he ascended into heaven, and sitteth at the right hand of God the Father Almighty; and from thence shall come again at the end of the world, to judge the quick and the dead? And dost thou believe in the Holy Ghost; the holy Catholick Church; the Communion of Saints; the Remission of sins; the Resurrection of the flesh; and everlasting life after death?

The sick person shall answer, All this I steadfastly believe.

Then shall the Minister examine whether he repent him truly of his sins, and be in charity with all the world; exhorting him to forgive, from the bottom of his heart, all persons that have offended him; and if he hath offended any other, to ask them forgiveness; and where he hath done injury or wrong to any man, that he make amends to the uttermost of his power. And if he have not before disposed of his goods, let him then be admonished to make his Will, and to declare his debts, what he oweth, and what is owing unto him; for the better discharging of his conscience, and the quietness of his Executors. But men should often be put in remembrance to take order for the settling of their temporal estates, whilst they are in health.

These words before rehearsed may be said before the Minister begin his Prayer, as he shall see cause. The Minister should not omit earnestly to move such sick persons as are of ability to be liberal to the poor.

Here shall the sick person be moved to make a special confession of his sins, if he feel his conscience troubled with any weighty matter. After which confession, the Priest shall absolve him (if he humbly and heartily desire it) after this sort.

OUR Lord Jesus Christ, who hath left power to his Church to absolve all sinners who truly repent and believe in him, of his great mercy forgive thee thine offences: And by his authority committed to me, I absolve thee from all thy sins, In the Name of the Father, and of the Son, and of the Holy Ghost. Amen.

And then the Priest shall say the Collect following.

Let us pray. O most merciful God, who, according to the multitude of thy mercies, dost so put away the sins of those who truly repent, that thou rememberest them no more: Open thine eye of mercy upon this thy servant, who most earnestly desireth pardon and forgiveness. Renew in him, most loving Father, whatsoever hath been decayed by the fraud and malice of the devil, or by his own carnal will and frailness; preserve and continue this sick member in the unity of the Church; consider his contrition, accept his tears, assuage his pain, as shall seem to thee most expedient for him. And for asmuch as he putteth his full trust only in thy mercy, impute not unto him his former sins, but strengthen him with thy blessed Spirit; and, when thou art pleased to take him hence, take him unto thy favour, through the mer-

Sickness: its Trials and Blessings

its of thy most dearly beloved Son Jesus Christ our Lord. Amen.

Then shall the Minister say this Psalms 71.

In thee, O Lord, have I put my trust: let me never be put to confusion: but rid me, and deliver me in thy righteousness; incline thine ear unto me, and save me.

Be thou my strong hold, where unto I may always resort: thou hast promised to help me; for thou art my house of defence, and my castle.

Deliver me, O my God, out of the hand of the ungodly: out of the hand of the unrighteous and cruel man.

For thou, O Lord God, art the thing that I long for: thou art my hope, even from my youth.

Through thee have I been holden up ever since I was born: thou art he that took me out of my mother's womb; my praise shall alway be of thee. I am become as it were a monster unto many: but my sure trust is in thee.

O let my mouth be filled with thy praise: that I may sing of thy glory and honour all the day long.

Cast me not away in the time of age: forsake me not when my strength faileth me.

For mine enemies speak against me, and they that lay wait for my soul take their counsel together, saying: God hath forsaken him, persecute him, and take him; for there is none to deliver him.

Go not far from me, O God: my God, haste thee to help me.

Let them be confounded and perish that are against my soul: let them be covered with shame and dishonour that seek to do me evil.

As for me, I will patiently abide alway: and will praise thee more and more.

Sickness: its Trials and Blessings

My mouth shall daily speak of thy righteousness and salvation: for I know no end thereof.

I will go forth in the strength of the Lord God: and will make mention of thy righteousness only.

Thou, O God, hast taught me from my youth up until now: therefore will I tell of thy wondrous works.

Forsake me not, O God, in mine old age, when I am grayheaded: until I have shewed thy strength unto this generation, and thy power to all them that are yet for to come.

Thy righteousness, O God, is very high, and great things are they that thou hast done: O God, who is like unto thee?

Glory be to the Father and to the Son: and to the Holy Ghost;

As it was in the beginning, is now, and ever shall be: world without end. Amen.

Adding this.

O Saviour of the world, who by thy Cross and precious Blood hast redeemed us, Save us, and help us, we humbly beseech thee, O Lord.

Then shall the Minister say,

The Almighty Lord, who is a most strong tower to all them that put their trust in him, to whom all things in heaven, in earth, and under the earth, do bow and obey, be now and evermore thy defence; and make thee know and feel, that there is none other Name under heaven given to man, in whom, and through whom, thou mayest receive health and salvation, but only the Name of our Lord Jesus Christ. Amen.

And after that shall say,

UNTO God's gracious mercy and protection we commit thee. The Lord bless thee, and keep thee. The Lord make his face to shine upon thee, and be gracious unto thee. The Lord lift

Sickness: its Trials and Blessings

up his countenance upon thee, and give thee peace, both now and evermore. Amen.

A Prayer for a sick Child

O Almighty God, and merciful Father, to whom alone belong the issues of life and death: Look down from heaven, we humbly beseech thee, with the eyes of mercy upon this child now lying upon the bed of sickness: Visit him, O Lord, with thy salvation; deliver him in thy good appointed time from his bodily pain, and save his soul for thy mercies' sake: That, if it shall be thy pleasure to prolong his days here on earth, he may live to thee, and be an instrument of thy glory, by serving thee faithfully, and doing good in his generation; or else receive him into those heavenly habitations, where the souls of them that sleep in the Lord Jesus enjoy perpetual rest and felicity. Grant this, O Lord, for thy mercies' sake, in the same thy Son our Lord Jesus Christ, who liveth and reigneth with thee and the Holy Ghost, ever one God, world without end. Amen.

A Prayer for a sick person, when there appeareth small hope of recovery.

O Father of mercies, and God of all comfort, our only help in time of need: we fly unto thee for succour in behalf of this thy servant, here lying under thy hand in great weakness of body. Look graciously upon him, O Lord; and the more the outward man decayeth, strengthen him, we beseech thee, so much the more continually with thy grace and Holy Spirit in the inner man. Give him unfeigned repentance for all the errors of his life past, and steadfast faith in thy Son Jesus; that his sins may be done away by thy mercy, and his pardon sealed in heaven, before he go hence, and be no more seen.

Sickness: its Trials and Blessings

We know, O Lord, that there is no word impossible with thee; and that, if thou wilt, thou canst even yet raise him up, and grant him a longer continuance amongst us: Yet, forasmuch as in all appearance the time of his dissolution draweth near, so fit and prepare him, we beseech thee, against the hour of death, that after his departure hence in peace, and in thy favour, his soul may be received into thine everlasting kingdom, through the merits and mediation of Jesus Christ, thine only Son, our Lord and Saviour. Amen.

A commendatory Prayer for a sick person at the point of departure

O Almighty God, with whom do live the spirits of just men made perfect, after they are delivered from their earthly prisons: We humbly commend the soul of this thy servant, our dear brother, into thy hands, as into the hands of a faithful Creator, and most merciful Saviour; most humbly beseeching thee, that it may be precious in thy sight. Wash it, we pray thee, in the blood of that immaculate Lamb, that was slain to take away the sins of the world; that whatsoever defilements it may have contracted in the midst of this miserable and naughty world, through the lusts of the flesh, or the wiles of Satan, being purged and done away, it may be presented pure and without spot before thee. And teach us who survive, in this and other like daily spectacles of mortality, to see how frail and uncertain our own condition is; and so to number our days, that we may seriously apply our hearts to that holy and heavenly wisdom, whilst we live here, which may in the end bring us to life everlasting, through the merits of Jesus Christ thine only Son our Lord. Amen.

Sickness: its Trials and Blessings

A Prayer for persons troubled in mind or in conscience

O Blessed Lord, the Father of mercies, and the God of all comforts: We beseech thee, took down in pity and compassion upon this thy afflicted servant. Thou writest bitter things against him, and makest him to possess his former iniquities; thy wrath lieth hard upon him, and his soul is full of trouble: But, O merciful God, who hast written thy holy Word for our learning, that we, through patience and comfort of thy holy Scriptures, might have hope; give him a right understanding of himself, and of thy threats and promises; that he may neither cast away his confidence in thee, nor place it any where but in thee. Give him strength against all his temptations, and heal all his distempers.

Break not the bruised reed, nor quench the smoking flax. Shut not up thy tender mercies in displeasure; but make him to hear of joy and gladness, that the bones which thou hast broken may rejoice. Deliver him from fear of the enemy, and lift up the light of thy countenance upon him, and give him peace, through the merits and mediation of Jesus Christ our Lord. Amen.

The Communion of the Sick

For as much as all mortal men be subject to many sudden perils, diseases, and sicknesses, and ever uncertain what time they shall depart out of this life; therefore, to the intent they may always be in a readiness to die, whensoever it shall please Almighty God to call them, the Curates shall diligently from time to time (but especially in the time of pestilence, or other infectious sickness) exhort their Parishioners to the often receiving of the holy Communion of the Body and Blood of our Saviour Christ, when it shall be publickly ministered in the Church; that so doing, they may, in case of sudden visitation, have the less cause to be disquieted for lack of the same. But if the sick person be not able to come to the Church, and yet is desirous to receive the Communion in his house; then he must give timely notice to the Curate, signifying also how many there are to communicate with him, (which shall be three, or two at the least,) and having a convenient place in the sick man's house, with all things necessary so prepared, that the Curate may reverently minister, he shall there celebrate the holy Communion, beginning with the Collect, Epistle, and Gospel, here following.

The Collect

Almighty, everliving God, Maker of mankind, who dost correct those whom thou dost love, and chastise every one whom thou dost receive: We beseech thee to have mercy upon this thy servant visited with thine hand, and to grant that he may take his sickness patiently, and re- cover his bodily health, (if it be thy gracious will;) and whensoever his soul shall depart from the body, it may be without spot presented unto thee; through Jesus Christ our Lord. Amen.

The Epistle. Heb 12. 5.

My son, despise not thou the chastening of the Lord, nor faint when thou art rebuked of him. For whom the Lord loveth he chasteneth; and scourgeth every son whom he receiveth.

The Gospel. St. John 5. 24.

Verily, verily I say unto you, He that heareth my word, and believeth on him that sent me, hath everlasting life, and shall not come into condemnation; but is passed from death unto life.

After which the Priest shall proceed according to the form before prescribed for the holy Communion, beginning at these words [Ye that do truly, &c.]

Sickness: its Trials and Blessings

At the time of the distribution of the holy Sacrament, the priest shall first receive the Communion himself, and after minister unto them that are appointed to communicate with the sick, and last of all to the sick person.

But if a man, either by reason of extremity of sickness, or for want of warning in due time to the curate, or for lack of company to receive with him, or by any other just impediment, do not receive the Sacrament of Christ's Body and Blood, the Curate shall instruct him, that if he do truly repent him of his sins, and stedfastly believe that Jesus Christ both suffered death upon the Cross for him, and shed his Blood for his redemption, earnestly remembering the benefits he hath thereby, and giving him hearty thanks therefore, he doth eat and drink the Body and Blood of our Saviour Christ profitably to his Soul's health, although he do not receive the Sacrament with his mouth.

When the sick person is visited, and receiveth the holy Communion all at one time, then the Priest, for more expedition, shall cut off the form of the Visitation at the Psalms [In thee, O Lord, have I put my trust &c] and go straight to the Communion.

In the time of the plague, sweat, or such other like contagious times of sickness or diseases, when none of the Parish or neighbours can be gotten to communicate with the sick in their houses, for fear of the infection, upon special request of the diseased, the Minister may only communicate with him.

Made in the USA
Lexington, KY
06 June 2013